Homeopathy

The Great Riddle

Homeopathy

The Great Riddle

Richard Grossinger

North Atlantic Books
Berkeley, California

Homeopathy: The Great Riddle

Published by
North Atlantic Books
P.O. Box 12327
Berkeley, California 94712

Cover art by Harry S. Robins
Cover design by Nancy Koerner
Book design by Paula Morrison
Printed in the United States of America

Homeopathy: The Great Riddle is sponsored by the Society for the Study of Native Arts and Sciences, a nonprofit educational corporation whose goals are to develop an educational and crosscultural perspective linking various scientific, social, and artistic fields; to nurture a holistic view of arts, sciences, humanities, and healing; and to publish and distribute literature on the relationship of mind, body, and nature.

Library of Congress Cataloging-in-Publication Data
Grossinger, Richard, 1944–
    Homeopathy : the great riddle / Richard Grossinger.
        p.   cm.
    Rev. ed. of: Homeopathy : an introduction for skeptics and
beginners / Richard Grossinger. 1993.
    Includes bibliographical references and index.
    ISBN 1-55643-290-9 (trade paper : alk. paper)
    1. Homeopathy. 2. Homeopathy—United States. 3. Hahnemann,
Samuel, 1755–1843. I. Title.
RX71.G78   1998
615.5'32—dc20   98-6345
                                                                                                CIP

1   2   3   4   5   6   7   8   /   02   01   00   99   98

Preface

There are many books on how to practice homeopathic medicine, its remedies and character types. This book, *Homeopathy: The Great Riddle,* is an attempt to understand what homeopathy is.

Defining homeopathy is not a simple matter. For one, it has no coherent physical, biochemical, or anatomical theory, at least by modern experimental standards. Homeopathy originates from an historical event at the close of the eighteenth century and has not been definitively reevaluated or updated since. It has rested solely, since then, on its apparent and mystifying success in curing serious and chronic diseases. Meanwhile, its language, science, and philosophy have remained in much the state they were at its inception despite monumental change in the rest of the world.

Chapter 2, "The Origins of Homeopathic Medicine," discusses the medical and pharmaceutical systems that preceded homeopathy and from which it assembled its methods and rationales. Without understanding prior systems that are similar to homeopathy, it is difficult to see how homeopathy arrived at its unusual tenets. Notably none of these other systems has survived intact into the present.

The core of this book is Chapter 3, "The Principles and Methodology of Homeopathic Medicine." In this section I have summarized the belief system behind homeopathy, pointing out both the ways in which it is convincing and the ways in which it is fantastic and requires a leap of faith. The major premises of homeopathic medicine cannot be concretized; thus, homeopathy must explain itself by a mixture of archaic and futuristic paradigms, ranging from alchemy to chaos theory. My purpose in this chapter is neither to acclaim nor refute homeopathy but to disclose its workings.

Chapter 4 reviews the discovery and development of homeopathy by Samuel Hahnemann and explains how the German physician codified a highly unorthodox healing system while fancying he was engaged in mainstream research.

Chapter 5 describes homeopathy's temporary triumph in nineteenth-century North America, followed by its almost total demise in the early years of the twentieth century, then its revival in the 1970s. The wave of scientific enthusiasm that made homeopathy the supreme American medicine at the time of the Civil War and in the decades thereafter changed direction in the early twentieth century and utterly dashed it. In a startlingly short period of time, homeopathy went from the most progressive and modern medicine known to man to a museum piece. Once laboratory science looked closely at homeopathy, Hahnemann's thesis seemed to unravel into folklore and superstition; it was quickly dismissed. Yet when the counterculture brought new paradigms into society (and healing), homeopathy was mercurially reborn.

Appendices include a case history and a comparison of homeopathy to other alternative and conventional medical systems.

Certain areas touched on in this book are covered in greater depth in my other writings.

Morphogenetic theories behind microdose activity are examined throughout my embryology book, *Getting Made: Species, Gender, and Identity* (North Atlantic Books, 1998).

Alchemical medicine is described in detail in an essay "Alchemy: Pre-Egyptian Legacy, Millennial Promise" in my anthology entitled *The Alchemical Tradition in the Late Twentieth Century* (North Atlantic Books, 1979, 1991).

The relation of homeopathy to other alternative medicines is explored throughout my two-volume work on the history and philosophy of medicine: *Planet Medicine: Origins* and *Planet Medicine: Modalities* (North Atlantic Books, 1996). In fact, a much briefer version of *Homeopathy: The Great Riddle* appeared in the early edition, *Planet Medicine: From Stone Age Shamanism to Post-Industrial Healing* (Doubleday Anchor, 1980; Shambhala Publications, 1982; North Atlantic Books, 1987, 1990). It was first published in its own volume in 1993 as *Homeopathy: An Introduction for Beginners and Skeptics* and then revised in 1998 into its present form.

Table of Contents

Foreword

by Dana Ullman, M.P.H.

Homeopathy is either a highly sophisticated method of stimulating placebo response, or it is a powerful, though mysterious, method of healing. Either way, homeopathic medicine is worthy of thorough investigation.

The evidence, both historical and scientific, put forth in this book strongly suggests that the placebo explanation is at best inadequate. Trying to explain the various phenomena witnessed and experienced from homeopathic medicines as simply a placebo response leads to a cheap, intellectually weak answer. Such simpleminded explanations suggest that the person has not done his or her homework and is unfamiliar with homeopathy's history and present status.

Homeopathy achieved its greatest popularity in the nineteenth century because of its successes in treating the infectious disease epidemics that raged during that time, including cholera, yellow fever, scarlet fever, and typhoid. Could one convincingly assume that this undeniable success was the result of a placebo?

Trying to explain the effects of homeopathic medicine as simply placebos ignores present-day experience as well. Homeopathy is used by 39 percent of practicing French physicians and 20 percent of German physicians. Over 40 percent of British physicians refer to homeopathic physicians, and 45 percent of Dutch physicians consider the medicines effective. Based on these statistics, homeopathy should not be considered "alternative medicine"; it is an integral part of mainstream health care. Could one convincingly assume that homeopathy would have this level of acceptance in the European medical community if the medicines were simply placebos?

And then there is the experimental evidence. There is a small but significant body of clinical and laboratory research that substantiates homeopathy. It is not the primary purpose of this book to cite or discuss in detail these studies, for Grossinger is more interested in the paradoxes that homeopathy creates and the dialogue that ensues than he is in the research itself. He is more interested in the philosophical, sociological, and anthropological implications of various modes of medical care. He revels and immerses himself in the mystery of the phenomenon of healing, and at the same time, he keeps a certain distance from all specific practices in order to take a long, hard, inquisitive view of the sometimes confusing, sometimes enlightening science and art of healing.

Grossinger is also sophisticated enough to realize that research on entities as complex as homeopathic medicines must be conducted in the context of their method of preparation and use. For instance, it is generally not possible to test homeopathic medicines without individualizing the medicines according to homeopathic principles. It is inadequate and inappropriate to test microdoses as if they were standardized drugs meant for everyone with the same symptoms.

Grossinger's account tells us why explaining homeopathy as simply placebo effect evades a consideration of the more profound questions that homeopathy raises vis-à-vis both science and society. What are the implications of such medicines on physics, chemistry, immunology, and health care? What are the implications of homeopathy for understanding disease, health, and the healing process?

Homeopathy, especially the energetic, spiritual nature of its medicines, is based on significantly different premises from those of conventional medicine and even from those of herbal medicine. Distinguishing homeopathy from the both the natural therapies that seek to purge and cleanse the body and the mechanistic, biomedical methods that directly attack the pathological processes in the human body, Grossinger notes how its vitalistic basis leads it to a unique perspective on disease and a radically different approach to treating it. This vitalistic perspective is at once ancient and futuristic, lying at the heart of most indigenous peoples' understanding of the human body as well as of most science fiction authors' description of energy fields (witness George Lucas' "Star Wars" trilogy and his leading characters oft-repeated "May the Force be with you").

Originally trained as an anthropologist, Grossinger seems to take a special pleasure in finding different ways to contrast modern medical culture (which is largely based on the prescription of crude doses of synthetic drugs) with the medical alchemy of homeopathy and other energy medicines.

To Grossinger, homeopathy integrates aspects of ancient medicine and the scientific method. I would add that although homeopathy itself was not formally systematized until the late 1700s and early 1800s by Dr. Samuel Hahnemann, its fundamental principle, the Law of Similars, was known and written about by Hippocrates, Paracelsus, and numerous others throughout Western history. Hahnemann's unique contribution to homeopathy's development was the use of provings, which are experiments in which a substance is given in continual crude or energetic doses until symptoms of overdose are elicited. Because these experiments have been employed since the origins of homeopathy to determine what symptoms a medicine is effective in treating, a form of controlled experimentation continues to lie at the basis of the homeopathic method. In fact, historians readily acknowledge that homeopathy in the nineteenth century was considerably more scientifically based than conventional medicine of that era.

Grossinger takes us on a journey through much of this history into our modern day. He invokes in turn various mysteries that homeopathy presents. Ultimately, he helps us ask more sophisticated questions about disease, health, and healing. Although readers may be better prepared to address these questions after reading this book, they will inevitably be humbled by yet more profound questions that continue to lie underneath.

—Berkeley, California
September 1993

Chapter 1

What is
Homeopathy?

Homeopathy was developed by the German physician Samuel Hahnemann (1755–1843) in the late eighteenth and early nineteenth centuries and quickly became a dominant medical practice in much of the Western world until the early twentieth century. Its ascent was greatest in North America, cresting during the decade from 1880 to 1890; its decline was most swift and thorough there, too. Briefly stated, as laboratory science took over medicine, homeopathy ran into its own insurmountable internal contradictions and ultimately lost its identity as a single consistent system. The policies of the American Medical Association and Abraham Flexner's *Report on Medical Education in the United States and Canada* (1910) finally undermined homeopathy's professional standing, and it was isolated as a nonscientific medicine. The old practitioners died in dishonor, and until a dramatic revival during the 1970s, hardly any young recruits took their places.

What is homeopathy? In a 1992 article in *The New York Times Magazine* James Gorman notes the confusion raised by the recent popularity of the system:

> Few people who buy the new over-the-counter homeopathic remedies realize that homeopathy is not herbal or Chinese medicine. It is not naturopathy, osteopathy or acupuncture, not bodywork, shiatsu or chiropractic.[1]

Homeopathy is first, and perhaps foremost, a continuation of the long empirical traditions of Western medicine. That is, its "science" and philosophy arise directly from the treatment of the sick, and historically its claims have been based more on results than on any demonstrable mode of healing. By today's reductionist definition it is not a science. Despite the arguments of some supporters that it is "another scientific medicine," we more likely could conclude that it is "the medicine of an unknown science."

Homeopathy contains elements of Vitalism, hermeticism, and early pharmacology, all conceived of simultaneously as part of one method. If we listen carefully to the homeopathic tune we hear echoes of these themes resonating through one another. In another sense, homeopathy is the only branch of hermetic science that has succeeded, if temporarily and incompletely, in gaining professional standing as a secular trade. That alone is a miracle.

Homeopathy is based theoretically on the responsiveness of the defense mechanism rather than the intercession of the physician. This defense mechanism is neither visible nor associated with any organ or system. It is intrinsic in the integrity of the organism, whether that integrity is understood as morphogenetic fields, elemental charge, or the interplay of yin and yang. It has the power to respond appropriately to any disease and thus is a direct descendant of the vital force of Greek and Mediaeval medicine and a derivative from the alchemy of Paracelsus and Van Helmont. In all such systems disease is an "invasive idea" superficially imposed upon an energetic restorative function at the heart of every life-form.

Homeopathy also makes a unique excursion into "Stone Age medicine," for it is holistic and dynamic in the same way that Navaho and Australian Aboriginal medicine are, though hardly for the same reasons. Homeopathy is clinical and detached, not shamanic or participatory. At a hypothetical "Cosmic Healing Conference," witch doctors and homeopaths would go at once to opposite sides of the room.

Homeopathy is neither the first nor the last attempt to develop a scientific Vitalist medicine. Alchemists, gnostics, animists, Rosicrucians, and other naturalist-magicians worked for prior millennia toward a cure based on the life force and the primal energy of nature. Goethe, Steiner, Jung, and Reich have followed. Homeopathy is notable, though, for its unlikely combination of elements and its time of birth. There seems no reason why it should have arisen when it did, at the turn of the nineteenth century, when the hermetic and magical sciences were in decline and the scientific revolution was building toward a crescendo. Surely, if there were a microdose principle of healing, the ancient Egyptians or Greeks would have come upon it, and Paracelsus would have incorporated it in his hermetic medicine. Why a new hermetic science at the very end of active occult research?

It would seem that if homeopathy had not been inherited by the Middle Ages, it would have skipped a few centuries for the quantum sciences of the future. Yet it appeared, no doubt for some profoundly appropriate reason, at a hiatus in magical-psychological inquiry, and it persists as a clinical occult discipline through this period before the full rebirth of paraphysical studies. It stands today as a singular, tantalizing clue to how we might address polluted oceans, deteriorating atmosphere, and spreading episodes of famine and plague.

Homeopathy, as we know it, is the invention of Samuel Hahnemann. One man's discoveries define it more thoroughly than the laws of Newton define physics. Although aspects of homeopathic thought were in existence before Hahnemann, the system itself arises as suddenly from his mind as Mormonism did from the golden tablets of Joseph Smith. Before Hahnemann, there was no homeopathy. Since Hahnemann, homeopathy has changed only to a minor degree, much less than biology and physics during the same time. To his supporters, Hahnemann is the single genius in the history of recorded medicine, if not the history of science. To his detractors, he is a bizarre case in the legacy of delusion.

It is a mistake to assume that homeopathy began as an unorthodox or even an alternative medical system. We tend to forget the different conditions into which it was born. In Hahnemann's day, medicine was in a formative phase; few theories or facts were firm. Mainstream practice relied almost entirely on procedures and drugs which today would be considered primitive, dangerous, and ineffective. Even a hundred years later, by the subsequent acknowledgment of doctors and historians, physicians stood an equal chance of harming or helping a patient.

Hahnemann was not a maverick by temperament; he intended only methodological reform of this dangerous mess, a reasonable contribution to the general research of his time. He assumed that he had discovered the same laws of cure that others were seeking, and that mainstream science would ultimately vindicate him.

The initial response to Hahnemann's work was not totally out of keeping with this expectation. This does not mean that he was received with open arms; in fact, he found himself in swift conflict with much of the medical profession. But he also had significant support, and the medicine of that time was already a hodgepodge of competing, combative beliefs. There was no regulatory body, medical or legal, to decide among interpretations, nor was there any generally agreed-upon principle of physics or chemistry that challenged homeopathy's (or any system's) claim to science. Hahnemann was one more candidate seeking a constituency. The resistance to him might have seemed official at times, but the rapid growth of Hahnemannism during and after his lifetime proves otherwise. Homeopathy lost some local battles, but it was not until the twentieth century that it was banished as an "imposter."

Hahnemann did not understand the revolutionary nature of what he was doing. He stumbled through a series of inexplicable experimental successes that led to a new set of meanings. His claims were so radical and their implications so far-reaching that, in truth, they could never be included in the mainstream of medical thought, not then, and not now. It is frankly absurd that today numerous homeopaths intend to see homeopathy accepted in general medical orthodoxy. Without revolutionary change at the very roots of science, homeopathy has no place among anatomy, chemistry, and general biology.

Clinical homeopathy cannot be verified even in the twentieth century's high-tech laboratory, which means, pessimistically, that scientific testing has already disproved *all* homeopathic claims. Many homeopaths would deny this, and they cite an array of experiments in the chemistry of enzymes, colloids, trace elements, hormones, and fractals. Some of this research is interesting and provocative, but it boils down to mere isolated events, without controlled retesting and certainly without orientation to the rest of science, nor does any of the research test the exact claims of homeopathic microdilution.

If we were to side with orthodoxy here, on the basis of the impossibility of homeopathic science, we would be left still with two significant events: one, the startling and repeated therapeutic success of hundreds of thousands of homeopathic physicians in all parts of the world for more than a century of practice, and two, a homeopathic attack on the methods and goals of mainstream medicine that does not require the acceptance of homeopathic principles for its validity.

Homeopathy has been defined in a variety of ways, and although most homeopaths will argue for a single orthodox version, nothing has marked the history of this medicine more than its own disagreements about what its rules are.

The fundamental split is between pure Hahnemannian homeopaths and later, more pragmatic adaptors. The purists insist on following their interpretation of Hahnemannian procedure scripturally and to the exclusion of all other methods. The pragmatists, on the other hand, continue to reinvent and modernize homeopathy and its language as the world changes. Ironically, Hahnemann himself was a purist only insofar as he proposed the various axioms on which homeopathic purism is based. Over his lifetime, Hahnemann repeatedly broke his own rules and replaced prior orthodoxies with new competing ones. In addition, his pursuits encompassed a number of realms that nowadays homeopaths would ignore or disdain. Hahnemannian medicine in its own era was not even initially homeopathy, let alone Hahnemannian homeopathy. That rigidity comes a century later from the use of the founder's writings to establish a new science based on inalterable principles of healing in nature.

Fundamentalist homeopaths have interpreted the progressive relationship of disease and civilization by laws of profound, incurable disease layers, while other homeopathic practitioners have dealt solely with patients. The result has been a growing discrepancy between treatments and their rationale.

Although Hahnemann invented the unique system we call "homeopathy," many of its elements were in existence in different dialects beforehand. Of particular note, the practice of giving a medicine that initially heightens symptomology (i.e., feeds the symptoms) had been around since prehistoric times and was an important part of Hippocratic and Paracelsian medicine.

Historically, prescribing a remedy with effects like those of the disease is known as the "Law of Similars." A doctor must choose both the right remedy and the moment of perfect fruition in the progression of a disease; otherwise the "cure" will not inspire or amplify coction (the body's natural conversion by heat). He must also distinguish between primary disease, which comes from the healthy reaction of the vital force (and can be treated by Similars), and secondary disease, which is really a sign of the capitulation of the patient's healing powers—often from the wrong treatment.

For instance, according to the principles of healing in early Hippocratic medicine, hemorrhages, hemorrhoids, nosebleed, diarrhea, and headaches were all signs that a disease was trying to work its way out and were encouraged. For an enlarged spleen, dysentery was considered progress. Diarrhea was usually interpreted as a ripening of white phlegm. Pain in the joints indicated that a fever was beginning to disperse. Varicose veins and hemorrhoids in an insane person were desirable consequences of the reentry of disease into the watery earthen body from the remote aery sphere where it was incurable.

On the other hand, angina followed by lung disease was a sign not of coction but the reverse: that rawness was taking over. Rashes were considered healthy (peptic), but not if one should disappear abruptly without some other corresponding improvement. Diarrhea, nosebleed, and expectoration were expected to provoke a crisis, with overall health following, or the disorder was thought to have settled deeper, with a weakening of the vital force.

In such traditions, however, the use of Similars as remedies was liberally mixed with the use of Contraries, and most doctors treated maladies on a shifting and subjective basis.

By basing homeopathy solely on the Law of Similars, Hahnemann formalized the distinction between a medicine that respects and encourages symptoms and all other medicines. He called the first, of course, "homeopathy" (from the Greek for "like treatment of disease") and the second "allopathy" (from the Greek for "other treatment of disease"). He meant to include in allopathy the medicine based on the supposed Law of Contraries, plus any other treatments that were not based on responding to symptomology with similar-acting medicines. Today, allopathy has become synonymous with the medical establishment, a word used not only pejoratively by homeopaths but proudly by physicians who have no sympathy for treatment by Similars. Yet these very doctors paradoxically encourage vaccinations to prevent disease and "identical" substances to cure allergies, methods more properly defined as isopathy (treating by the same). The contemporary homeopathic writer Dana Ullman shows homeopathic "patriotism" of the right Similars when he declares dismissively:

> Some conventional medical treatments are ultimately [also] based on the Law of Similars, though they should not be considered homeopathic medicines for two basic reasons: 1) each medicine is not prepared in the pharmacological procedure of dilution and succussion common to homeopathic medicines; 2) each medicine is not individually prescribed in the sufficient detail common to homeopathic medicines.
>
> A homeopathic medicine is not prescribed for a specific disease *per se*, but for the pattern of symptoms that it is known to cause in overdose when given to healthy people. The concept of pattern or syndrome of symptoms is an integral part of homeopathic care. This is simply a systems concept of looking at symptoms in context with the whole. The challenge to the person prescribing homeopathic medicines then is this individualization of drug prescription.[2]

We will return to these important matters later.

Hahnemann, as noted, did not imagine himself the inventor of a whole esoteric system; he regarded his work as general medicine, to which he made many contributions, of which homeopathy was initially only one. But at the time he presented his ideas and through-out most of the nineteenth century, the full body of Hahnemann-ian thought was considered homeopathy. Much of this lexicon, however, dealt with diet, hygiene, immunization, the preparation of medicines, and even the origin of germs and techniques of surgery (anti-homeopathic topics).

At the same time, nineteenth-century allopathy, with its leeches and mercury medicines, bore little resemblance to current allopathy which is actually a mixture of traditional Western beliefs, break-throughs during the nineteenth and twentieth centuries, and the long European tradition of experiment. The innovations that define modern allopathy came from American laboratory science and ear-ly twentieth-century British medicine; in addition, Hahnemann's non-homeopathic therapeutics were adopted almost in total by the establishment and remain a crucial aspect of allopathy (so much so that allopathic medical facilities are named after him). Only his homeopathic principles were "invalidated" and dropped from gen-eral practice.

The subsequent twentieth-century division into allopathy and homeopathy worldwide is the outcome of the concerted profes-sional scourging of microdose techniques and Similars from general medicine over seventy-five years. Although from a homeopath's point of view this has resembled a witch hunt, the attack on home-opathy is actually only a footnote to complete restandardization of medicine. In its struggle for consistency and accountability, medical convention either did away with or adapted any alternative method or technique—homeopathic, osteopathic, herbal, or other. Most people today know nothing of either homeopathy or allopathy: there are just doctors.

Medicine is a general global tradition with some homeopathic and isopathic elements. Homeopathy had its heyday before this stan-dardization and as a different system from the one it presently is, with a wider range of practices and a less rigid ideology. It was arguably America's first great medical fad. By the Civil War, home-opaths were more numerous, wealthier, and more popular than allopaths and maintained a network of prestigious medical schools and hospitals. Through their joint efforts with other sectarian healers, bloodletting and dosing with mercury were successfully criticized and eliminated. Hahnemann's hygiene and theories of pharmacy played a large role in the modernization of treatment. Only after mainstream medicine adopted a full range of reforms, many suggested by Hahnemann, was it equipped to ungratefully dismiss specific homeopathic procedure.

Although homeopathy did finally succumb to a no-holds-barred attack by the American Medical Association backed by the pharmaceutical companies, its inherent position was untenable anyway and it was splitting from within. Even many homeopathic physicians viewed themselves simply as doctors and came not to distinguish between homeopathy and allopathy, adopting new procedures and drugs as they appeared on the market and generally participating in technological progress. They held the old ideal of universal medicine without a corresponding commitment to homeopathy as the prime candidate, so they strayed without knowing it and without any clear certainty as to what was pure homeopathy and what was violation. Even Hahnemann's writings were not decisive on major issues, and in any case, progressive health care was a more attractive paradigm than the Law of Similars to most physicians. All therapeutic systems dissolved into the momentum of this revolutionary world-view fueled by technology.

Then, experimental science sided strongly and fatally (for homeopathy) with the allopaths. That is, it sided with the physics and chemistry that allopathy had come to use primarily in its diagnosis and treatments and by which it defined itself. As science set the guidelines for accountability in medicine, homeopathy was considered not accountable, hence unethical. Its theories offered no demonstrable sequence of cause and effect.

Many homeopaths accepted this fatal verdict and joined the mainstream. They did not want to be considered quacks, nor did they want to lose their claim to the cutting edge of science. A decade into the twentieth century, homeopathy was marginal medicine. To practice it by itself meant serious economic sacrifice. It was an expensive and time-consuming problem for homeopaths to gain both AMA credentials for practicing medicine (the M.D. license) and the education necessary for practicing homeopathy. It was not long before being a doctor of homeopathy had about the same standing as being an alchemist. Yet a bare moment of history had passed since homeopathy's widest acceptability. That is because most homeopaths bought the unchallenged verdict of the opposition and jumped ship, or had jumped ship unintentionally because they did not know the difference between homeopathy and any other medicine.

Today, for the first time, the difference between homeopathy and allopathy is a pure difference of medicinal principle. No side issue clouds this any longer. We have a choice.

If Hahnemann were to view the present situation, he would find not only that his great discovery had been abandoned and rejected beyond his worst fears, but also that he had succeeded. With some of modern medicine he would not be at odds. It has developed a system of controlled laboratory experiments, and it has come to a clearmindedness of scientific procedure. Hahnemann might discern what we do: that homeopathy was never actually defeated within the clinical realm, but by what chemists and biologists chose to agree on and, as the lawmakers of the scientific community, imposed on all systems purporting to be science.

The homeopathy of today, which has been revived as an alternative medicine, is not the original homeopathy, which was part of the general eighteenth- and nineteenth-century search for principles of diagnosis and cure. Only those parts of Hahnemannism left out of mainstream medicine are now called homeopathy.

Before antibiotics and medical specialization, homeopathy was proposed as a revolutionary new discovery, and it was heralded or vilified for years as "The New School." Today homeopathy struggles between datedness and futurism, under one aegis attempting to propose the unknown quantum science and parapsychology that will vindicate its laws rejected by physics and biology, and under another aegis attempting to reestablish Hahnemann's original orthodoxy and archaic characterology.

Chapter Two

The Origins of
Homeopathic Medicine

There are few systems that break so sharply with their predecessors that they seem the invention of a single individual. In recent times we consider Sigmund Freud's model of the unconscious mind and Albert Einstein's theory of relativity both radical departures from anything which came before them. Charles Darwin and Karl Marx also changed human reality to such a degree that a gap formed between the landscape brought into being by their visions and the world they inherited. What sparked the collective alteration of perception was not *primarily* novel information (like the magnified image of a chromosome or quasar), for in each instance we can trace the roots of the paradigm far back into history. It was a rearrangement of familiar ideas in a manner that revealed an undisclosed side of all of them at once.

Intuition of the unconscious mind is as old as the paintings on the cave walls at Lascaux—in fact, tens of thousands of years older . . . as old as language—but Freud reified the unconscious process when he fused it with models from anatomy, animal behavior, and social theory. Such a notion could not have existed before the West learned of the indigenous peoples of Africa and America; before theories of jurisprudence reconsidered the disposition of madness; and likely not before the true scale of the night sky and the cell began to seep into philosophy. Suddenly one neurologist realized that our thought processes represent but a minute portion of our mental activity and that the nervous system binds an enormous nonconscious portion by the same phenomenology that shapes personalities and society.

Coming a century earlier and likewise the grand synthesis of one man, homeopathy foreshadowed psychiatry—not in its overall organization of meaning but in its concern for the interdynamics of mental and physical symptoms and its attempt to establish a code for the psychosomatic expression of the whole organism. Samuel Hahnemann took the sum of medical theory up to his time, reconceived it, and provided an alternative interpretation and synthesis. While his goals were modest, he invented a science not only of medicine but of psychology and physics. Whether this was an authentic set of laws or a bizarre metaphysical fantasy is not the sole issue: its sheer persistence is an indication that homeopathic inquiry is an unintegrated aspect of our understanding of nature in general and disease and healing in particular.

The divergence of cultural acceptability between homeopathy and psychiatry is also notable. Whereas psychiatry was able to become a well-bred and educated statesman and translate its primitive cryptography into a workable academic theory, homeopathy has remained a whirling dervish on the outskirts of science. Psychiatry works as logical materialism; homeopathy is disjunctive and paraphysical.

In order to understand Hahnemann's medical legacy, we must disinter an ancient rivalry between two informal lineages of doctors. On one side, beginning no doubt in Palaeolithic times with massage therapists, anatomical craftspeople, and herbalists, are the guilds of bonesetters, surgeons, and pharmacists. Their tools passed naturally from clan to clan and generation to generation over tens of thousands of years, then into the first civilizations in the form of accumulated knowledge and customs. In ancient and mediaeval epochs, these practical healers allied with barbers and smiths, but as university training and formal philosophy became prerequisites for medical practice, they isolated themselves from the more menial crafts as well as from the lay practice of energy healing. By the twentieth century, they had become the medical profession. They achieved that status primarily as an academic cult and a trade union, not in the lineage of their empirical forerunners.

The rivals of these professional doctors, friendly or aloof, collaborating or uninvolved, were shamans, street healers, and charismatic magicians. As shamans, they blended spiritual potions and called upon transcendental forces. As doctor-priests, they drew on a legacy of witchcraft and herbalism. As lay physicians, they treated their patients by a variety of means, always setting the goal of cure above explanations and theories (though many of them had theories—religious, proto-scientific, animistic, Vitalistic, etc.). Early in recorded history, they were indistinguishable from doctors; in fact, they often *were* the doctors and combined both modalities of medicine. A shaman could be a spiritual healer and a surgeon, a Vitalist and a pharmaceutical herbalist, without being aware that there was even a distinction or opposition between the two. The personae were practiced almost like alternating totem masks; even where they were not joined in the personality of one "medicine man," they were in essential balance and alliance. It was only very gradually, as objectified science protruded, that these healers, as a class, took leave of the credentialed medicine guild. From Chinese, Ayurvedic, and Druid medical visionaries and apothecaries to Greek and Roman philosophers, there is a gap in epistemology.

Homeopathy is one possible outcome, centuries later, of the dialectic between these two traditions. A "scientific," laboratory medicine, it is still based on intuitive, holistic diagnoses, spiritualized herbs and minerals, and the Law of Similars rather than on academic anatomy and pharmacy.

In his four-volume history of medicine, *Divided Legacy*, Harris Coulter defines an "Empirical tradition" of healing: diagnosing patients from careful observation, interpreting symptoms as signs of deeper holistic changes, and developing a practical compendium of wisdom from the actual treatment of the sick. This was opposed from the time of early Greece by a so-called "Rationalist tradition," which was based on the use of anatomical and pharmacological logic to develop unchallengeable cause-and-effect etiologies of disease and cure. Disease-as-entity, taxonomy of disease, gave rise to a science of pathology.

A Rationalist seeks a general theory explaining the diverse elements and curative actions that may have been successful in individual treatments. Laws of healing, which are laws of nature, take precedent over single cures. The methods of modern orthodox medicine, refined over centuries, are, in essence, applications of cause and effect from models of biomechanical action. "Empirical" medicine, however, eschews such laws as mirages based on abstractions. The Empiricist goes from case to case, developing an intuitive art and trying only to cure sick individuals. He places less value on authoritative medical knowledge because he believes each person is an irreducible whole. To him there are no categories of disease, only people who are sick and healers to read their distinctive shadings of pathology and cure. Homeopathy is the epitome of empirical medicine.

Where a Rationalist may jump on a symptom, such as bloody stools, and its likely cause, an Empiricist sees a codon with a variety of possible causes and interpretations depending on its placement and stage in a particular disease sequence. One of the authors of the library of information we know as the Hippocratic Corpus summarized this principle of diagnosis at least as far back as the fifth century BC: "Men are not feverish merely through heat. . . . the truth being that one and the same thing is both bitter and hot, or acid and hot, or salt and hot, with numerous other combinations, and cold again combines with other *dynameis*. It is these things which cause the harm. Heat, too, is present, but merely as a concomitant, having the strength of the directing factor which is aggravated and increases with the other factor. . . ."[1]

Insofar as a symptom is the result of the organism's immune response, neutralizing it in a misguided endeavor to reduce the damage it is causing may actually stifle and oppose the natural healing. Medicines chosen empirically according to the Law of Similars bolster coction by providing a push in the same direction. They are almost always the correct prescription.

Since coction is natural and performed by the body's intrinsic capacity for health, the doctor's job is to recognize and foster this process. Because Rationalist laws of cure linearize and simplify sequences of cause and effect, physicians practicing them overlook the far-reaching and holistic effects of any remedy; thus they spark an ever-present danger of new disease caused by their treatments themselves, especially where these counter and quell the immune response as if it were the disease. The illusion that one can ever limit an attack on selected symptoms to those loci alone has reached a *reductio ad absurdum* in the Rationalist's current overenthusiastic spectrum of antibiotics which can spawn long-term side-effects in individuals and also provide toxic environments for breeding more resistant germs by mutations, viral and bacterial recombinations, and natural selection.

Not all Empiricists are Vitalists. Even those who are do not share interpretations of the vital force. The spirits and voodoo powers of the shamans are, as we have noted, as much foolishness to most acupuncturists and homeopaths as they are to surgeons. Many faith healers and parapsychologists, on the other hand, accept the existence of telepathy or telekinesis without believing in the vital properties of plants and minerals, properties essential to the rationales of homeopathy, anthroposophical medicine, and alchemy.

Not all Vitalists are Empiricists, either. Nonempirical Vitalists have long entertained us with spiritualized energies and auras, most of which are proposed as having a universal basis in some transdimensional physics. Their advocates place them in the textbooks of anatomy and pharmacy, adding luminous grids of etheric and astral bodies to bones and nerve nets. Conversely, as modern psychiatry has proven, Rationalism can give rise to schools as characterological and intuitive as any ancient Empiricism. Homeopathy is unique in being both highly empirical and vitalistic, a quality it shares with Chinese medicine, Ayurveda, and some forms of osteopathy. Homeopathy has the fewest Rationalist elements that are nonvitalistic among all of these.

Whereas Empirical interpretations and methods probably represented the pre-fifth-century BC core of the Hippocratic Corpus, Rationalism appears to have flourished among a slightly later group of physicians associated historically with the Cnidians. Their treatments by opposites are familiar to us still. If there is fever, it must be lowered. If there is diarrhea, the physician should attack its dissipating cause. Pus in the lungs must be drained. Drugs and herbs are all presumed to work on a piecemeal humoral basis without the priority and holism of the vital force. If a person's system has accumulated undue wetness, a drying agent is added. If there is excess of heat, a cooling remedy is administered.

The Greek Rationalists were obsessed with figuring out how the body functioned—with an emphasis on chemicomechanical properties. By the time of Aristotle, abstract classification was beginning to circumscribe reality. Insofar as the data of sense perception were now distinguished from formal categories, diseases came to be seen as actual entities rather than as unknown patterns marked by combinations of perceptible symptoms. As this taxonomy became more sophisticated and confident, only those symptoms viewed as contributing directly to pathology were assigned value; the rest were either ignored or deemphasized. The disease became a discrete thing, named and tracked according to precedent. The "human body" of the Alexandrian physician Erasistratos (born around 300 BC) was a mere robot, a porous machine processing food and air as corpuscles. Digestion ground up matter and supplied the organs much in the manner of a simple mill. Basing their remedies on such models, Cnidian physicians prescribed scientifically, giving chemical solutions to neutralize toxic states, arouse sluggish organs, and dissolve specific congestions, respectively. When they found pus in the lungs, kidneys, or elsewhere, they aborted coction in an attempt to extract the accused pathogen. Later in history, with sharper knives, they excised the diseased tissue itself.

By contrast, as we have seen, the Empirical physician considered a rash a favorable sign, for it marked the progression of a disease outward from the core. However, if skin eruptions were not accompanied by general systemic improvement, they were an indication that the underlying pathology had abandoned its favored outlet and deepened. A new course was followed.

Empirical remedies were administered with a goal of aiding evacuation. "The aim of therapy is to assist the organism to combat the disease along the lines already selected by the organism; the medicines and techniques employed to this end may be described as operating on the basis of 'similarity' in that they stimulate the organism to continue along the path which it has already chosen."[2] Thus, herbs promoting heat might be given in a fever; cold baths might be prescribed for a chill.

Tracking the paths and stages of symptoms was the heart of empiricism: "Diseases cure themselves from the inside to the outside, the process of cure involves the appearance of new symptoms. . . . [The Empiricists sought] cure through spontaneous evacuation of the *materies morbi*, fever and sweating [considered] as favorable prognostic signs [with] the general idea that disease is resolved through an eruption or evacuation, with consequent suppuration or empyema if the evacuation is not complete."[3]

Since it was crucial to encourage the exiting of disease—and the coction which catalyzed it—the Empiricist's rule was: "Do not disturb a patient either during or just after a crisis, and try no experiments, neither with purges nor with other irritants, but leave him alone."[4] The doctor had to step aside.

Whereas the Rationalist tended to fill his ledgers with species of disease, like exotic plants and animals, and to spring upon his match with the indicated cure, the Empiricist waited and observed, staying true to the notion of a unique disease complex within an individual corresponding to the single force of coction. The appearance of multiple "diseases" was considered to represent different stages of life, variations of coction, or perhaps idiosyncratic constitutions: "Cheese does not harm all men alike; some eat their fill of it without the slightest hurt, nay, those it agrees with are wonderfully strengthened thereby. Others come off badly. So the *physies* of these men differ, and the difference lies in the constituent of the body which is hostile to cheese, and is aroused and stirred to action under its influence. . . . But if cheese were bad for the human *physis* without exception, it would have hurt all."[5]

The most innovative Empirical physician of Alexandrian times was Herophilos of Chalcedon who, among other things, charted the courses of diseases through a connection he perceived between the cycles of the *physis* and the rhythm of the pulse. "He developed a body of pulse doctrine in which pulse rates were classified according to size, speed, strength, rhythm, order, disorder, and irregularity. To make this knowledge graphic he based it on analogies with musical rhythms. He also compared various pulses to the movements of the gazelle, the ant, and the worm."[6] Diagnosis through pulse-taking has also been a mainstay of the highly empirical medicines of the Orient, though not of homeopathy.

As Roman science enveloped the Hippocratic Corpus, the new scientific Rationalists became even more mechanical, viewing coction as a mere abstraction. Conversion by bodily heat was cumbersome, indefinable, and—if it existed at all—cast only tantalizing ambiguities about which direction it might be going (healthy or morbid) and what doctors could do heroically to aid it. A medicine of similars was indirect and problematic by comparison with a medicine of contraries in which they could simply administer a neutralizing agent and produce the "miracle" of physician-assisted cure. A new mode of thinking evolved, which favored intellectual shortcuts to diagnosis and treatment and, most happily, quick results. Medicine was no longer an art but a rule-bound profession with favored treatments. Ultimately the practitioners of this profession adopted a sophisticated derivative of Erasistratos' anatomy: an animated corpse operating by mechanical laws, translating food and air into flesh and movement by the breakdown and rearrangement of raw materials. Coction was still invoked—it was the ghost or divinity behind healing—but there was an ongoing ambition to resolve it ultimately in terms of the mechanics of heat, moisture, and dissolution—as digestion and internal chemistry—which was considered a refinement, not a downgrading, of its original meaning. This was yet another step away from prehomeopathic thought.

In its most extreme form, Rationalism became Methodism, with all organic activity, including mind, viewed as the result of chance interactions of atoms. The Roman Methodist school of the Greek physicians Themison and Thessalus proposed the body as a porous pipe through which fluids circulate, too fast if the pipe is over-relaxed, too slow if it is too restricted. Sweating and bloodletting were the standard cures for a restricted flow, whereas darkness, quiet, and a diet of thick porridge and soft-boiled eggs constituted the remedy for agitated flow. Doctors began to lose a sense of whether their treatments were successful and to worry more about whether they fit established categories and traditional stages. Coulter points out "the 'fallacy of misplaced concreteness,' of [the physician] thinking he knows something about the organism when he has given names to its imaginary components."[7] The gap within medicine widened. Even as the Rationalists heralded vivisection and dissection as the ultimate tools in pinning down the proximate causes of illness, the Empiricists rejected the possibility of learning anything about health and disease from the quantitative analysis of corpses and laboratory experiments. As the first-century Roman physician Aulus Cornelius Celsus concluded: "All that is possible to come to know in the living, the actual treatment exhibits."[8] Celsus also wrote: "Nor is anything more foolish . . . than to suppose that whatever the condition of the part of a man's body in life, it will also be the same when he is dying, nay, when he is already dead . . . it is only when the man is dead that the chest and any of the viscera come into the view of the medical murderer, and they are necessarily those of a dead, not of a living man."[9] Yet the science of anatomy was leading in a direction from which Hahnemann would have to backtrack all the way to Celsus.

In spite of the fad of Rationalism, Celsus maintained the Empirical tradition during Roman times. Coulter cites some of his contributions:

> Madness is relieved by the formation of varicose veins, by dysentery, or by bleeding hemorrhoids. The cause of epileptic fits can be discharged through the stools. Watering of the eyes is benefited by diarrhoea. Shoulder pains spreading to the shoulder-blades or hands are relieved by a vomit of black bile. Prolonged diarrhoeas are suppressed by vomiting. . . . Dysentery benefits enlarged spleen. . . . Round worms in the stool at the disease crisis are a good sign. If bleeding hemorrhoids are suppressed, a sudden and serious disease is liable to supervene. . . .[10]

Celsus was clearly loyal to the Law of Similars:

He calls for black hellebore in disease where black bile is present, white hellebore in disease with white phlegm, and ox spleen as a remedy for enlarged spleen. Embedded splinters are drawn to the surface by a poultice made of pole-reed because "of splinters the pole-reed is the worst because it is rough. . . ." Likewise, "the scorpion is the best remedy against itself. Some pound up the scorpion and swallow it in wine; some pound it up in the same way and put it upon the wound; some put it upon a brazier and fumigate the wound with it. . . ." The remedy for an earache with maggots is oil in which maggots have been boiled. Hydrophobia was treated by throwing the patient into a pond.[11]

It is not only homeopathy that is portended here, although homeopathy is the most obvious inheritor of this tradition; it is the whole domain of sympathetic medicine, including the unwindings (*into* distortions) of osteopathy, the participatory traumas of gestalt psychoanalysis, and the warrior trainings of therapeutic aikido and other martial arts that transform fear by engaging its object.

The second-century Roman physician Galen was the vintage Rationalist. Son of a wealthy family in Pergamon (Asia Minor), he was extremely well educated, studying as a teenager with Aristotelians, Platonics, Stoics, and Epicureans. At twenty he went to Alexandria for eight years, completing his education. After serving four years as physician to the gladiators of Pergamon, he set out for Rome at the age of thirty-two. There he distinguished himself for both arrogance and superior knowledge, clearly the dominant doctor of his epoch.

Galen summarized the entire body of medicine that preceded him. His thirty or so volumes of writing (twenty surviving) represent the crucible for the development of medicine in the West. In the absence of any general theory of therapeutics, they served as the source of authority, partly by the sheer weight of their scholarship and partly because they had no rival. Whereas Galen did not favor fanatically mechanical Methodism, he supported the Rational approach and set it as the bellwether of medical knowledge for fourteen hundred years. More precisely, he attempted to meld all the different techniques and philosophies into one essential logos that brought together coction, *physis, dynameis,* and the various laws of cure. In doing this, almost unintentionally, he endowed the organs with a unique level of categorical existence by assigning to them powers in the form of *dynameis.* For the stomach, this was its digestive power, for the heart pulsation, for veins blood-making. Additionally, each of the organs encompassed four primal *dynameis:* attraction, retention, alteration, and expulsion.

Despite his seeming acknowledgment of vital power in the organs, Galen separated them from their organismic whole by giving them heterogeneous capacities. Coction was ultimately defined as the dynamic interplay of the four elements obeying the law of contraries. "Bodies act upon and are acted upon by each other in virtue of the Hot, Cold, Moist, and Dry. And if one is speaking of any activity, whether it be exercised by the veins, liver, arteries, heart, alimentary canal, or any part, one will be inevitably compelled to acknowledge that this activity depends upon the way in which the four qualities are blended."[12] Healing by supplying the lacking elemental quality is a determinate step toward a system that provides vitality only from outside the organism.

Galenic medicine, along with the Arabic versions of Avicenna, Rhazes, and Averroes that were based on it, remained dominant within a stagnant European medical tradition that became more and more isolated and provincial during the Middle Ages. The Empirical tradition stayed alive mainly as folk medicine. In fact, this essential dichotomy has persisted. Although formal medicine has burst out of the Galenic bubble as explosively as cosmology has broken out of the Ptolemaic universe, the Roman puzzle of the universe is still our reference point and, more importantly, our unacknowledged theoretical boundary.

The most notable break in the fourteen-hundred-year rule of Galenism in the direction of homeopathy was instigated by the Swiss physician Theophrastus Bombast von Hohenheim (1493–1541), who took on the name of Paracelsus not only to honor Celsus but to indicate that he had gone beyond him:

> I found the medicine which I had learned was faulty, and that those who had written about it neither knew nor understood it.

They all tried to teach what they did not know. They are vain-glorious babblers in all their wealth and pomp, and there is not more in them than in a worm-eaten coffin. So I had to look for a different approach.[13]

Such a quest led Paracelsus, by his own account, through Spain, Portugal, England, Germany, Prussia, Poland, Hungary, Transylvania, Croatia, Italy, and France; passing from village to village and region to region, he interviewed midwives and herbalists, bathkeepers and magicians, doctors and philosophers, priests and knights. His heroic ethnography alone restored the lost medical tradition by recovering its dispersed pieces. "What a doctor needs is not eloquence or knowledge of language and of books, illustrious though they be, but profound knowledge of nature and her works. . . . I do not compile from the excerpts of Hippocrates or Galen. In ceaseless toil I created them anew upon the foundation of experience. . . ."[14]

Although Paracelsus proposed a wide range of treatments, his emphasis upon the Doctrine of Similars was axiomatic:

"Never a hot illness has been cured by something cold, or a cold one by something hot. But it has happened that like has cured like."[15] This meant prescriptions as literal as sponge, crab's eyes, and *lapis lazuli* for calcareous deposits (tartar) in the body.

Paracelsus scorned the search for disease etiologies and matching remedies. By his theory the body exists only as the simultaneous activity of all its healthy members; hence, an illness occurs as a holistic spiritual entity, not just a disturbance in one locale where it is randomly noted or where it evidences the most pathology: "How then can the physician look for the maladies in the humors and assign their origins to them, since they are produced by the malady and not the malady by them? The snow doesn't make the winter, but the winter the snow. . . ."[16]

Because of his early years in the mines, he was sensitive to the mineral and alchemical basis of scourge and emphasized that the ailments of miners "are a spiritual entity caused by an emanation from the metal."[17] The actual symptoms act like a mild form of metal poisoning and can be healed only by encouraging the beneficial rather than pathological aspect of each metal in a medicine.

Paracelsus refused to categorize pathologies or seek exotic contraries to reverse their effects. Local conditions responsible for diseases always provided cures, as long as one had the perspicacity to recognize them. "Nothing else needs to be known to you in order to understand the matter, *corpus*, etc., of the disease than what the natural things of the earth and the elements indicate to you. If now you know the same, then you know the illness. Herein lies the anatomy, herefrom follows the medicine. For the medicine grows like the illness, and same and same yield each other's theory."[18]

Insofar as the beneficial similar of the metal in a medicine drives out its toxic emanation in a miner's body, a general formula for deriving remedies from plants and animals can be extrapolated (see below). Poisons have a particular role in this pharmacy because they are already potentized: "Consider, a spider is the supreme poison, on the other hand, also, the highest *arcanum* in chronic fevers."[19]

For centuries alchemists had sought the Quintessence of mercury and/or antimony in their attempts to synthesize the Philosopher's Stone and make gold. In his guise as proto-chemist, Paracelsus developed equivalent remedies not ordinarily associated with herbalism; that is, he sought to demonstrate that laboratory transmutation can turn animal, vegetable, and mineral substances into their Quintessences. Through a precise sequence of physical and spiritual stages involving decanters, ovens, invocations, and prayers, the alchemist-healer raises each raw potency through a new body that renders it active. Paracelsus' magical chemistry is reflected nowadays in contemporary alchemy and anthroposophical medicine rather than in homeopathy (which deals more purely with Similars than transmutation—and extracts essence by a different process).

There are, however, strong correspondences between Paracelsus' alchemy and Hahnemann's homeopathy: substances that in their crude state normally have no effect on the body—and certainly no medicinal effect—take on medicinal power when extracted and potentized into their "Quintessence." Thus, both alchemists and homeopaths liberate the curative aspects of common and simple substances; both are involved in the magical transmutation of matter into energy. Additionally, since the modality of alchemical medicine is spiritual, it is often the case that one drop is as good as a hundred drops; half a drop or even a fraction of a drop may be powerful enough. In some conditions, just the smell may be sufficient, for the whole of the Quintessence of the medicine works on the vital force of the organism. Homeopathy likewise produces medicines that become active on the basis of a single archetypal message rather than a commodity of digestible substance.

Whereas traditional Empirical medicine (and later, homeopathy) emphasized the Law of Similars, Paracelsus made elemental Hippocratic diagnosis only a part of his cosmology and added another, more astrally based iconography of selecting medicines according to "signatures" resembling the diseases they were to cure: "Whereas things to come may thus be known before in the Elements, by that wherein the Evesters dwell; some Evesters will be in the water, some in looking glasses, some in crystalls, some in polished muskles; some will be known by the commotions of waters, some by songs and by the mind."[20]

Signatures could be anything from color of minerals to places where plants grow, but are usually shapes of one or another part of a plant (hepatica for liver disease, walnut for ailments of the brain, St. John's wort for bruises and wounds because of the holes on its leaves resembling pores, aconite for eye diseases because its seed is small, dark, and round and contained in a white cuticle, etc.). Paracelsus explained: "As nature prefigures to us externally the mineral's nature in the rushes, in woods, and other plants, accordingly we shall also know that the salt in the body by its operation gives similar forms; from which it now follows that like heals its like, which is to say, equals form equal kinds of holes. And it has been shown with all types of holes that its like form has been its like medicine. Therefore it behooves the physician to know the anatomy of matching one thing with another."[21]

The Paracelsan physician Oswald Croll provided a supporting liturgy: "Magically, Plants through their Signatures speak to the man of medicine who looks deep within, and they manifest their Insides, hidden in the secret silence of Nature, to him through their likeness: for there is . . . a means of demonstration through likeness, a means by which the Great Demiurge is used to manifesting things divine and occult so that they yield up the supreme likeness of ideas. . . . All plants, flowers, trees, and other things coming forth from the earth are Books and Magical Signs, communicated by the enormous mercy of God, wherein those Signs may be our Medicine. . . ."[22]

Croll proclaims an esoteric and religious treasure hunt among cryptographs set in nature by a divine being. It is the medicine of astrology.

To trust such interpretations of divine puzzles may be risky, so Paracelsus provides an escape from doctrinal symbolism. Although the signature may lead the physician to the medicine, it is only through "testing" the substance that the properties suggested by the signature can be ensured. Homeopathy later added formal "proving" to the Law of Similars, but it disdained signatures as superstitions until the 1940s when Edward Whitmont suggested a possible system of morphological synchronicities (see pages 81–87).

The legacy of Paracelsus turned out to be a pantheon uniting macrocosm and microcosm, anatomy, pharmacology, the Doctrine of Signatures, the Law of Similars, etc., but the concordance was so vast for its time (like a cosmic field theory and a practical medicine joined) that it immediately fractured into alchemy, chemistry, herbalism, pharmacology, hermetic philosophy, and magic in the hands of his different followers. As Paracelsan alchemy merged with conventional pharmacy, it lost the Doctrine of Signatures and the astrological botany twinning plants and stars. At the same time, the specific medicines became so immediately popular that Paracelsan chemists virtually took over the drugstores of central Europe, their influence later spreading to the court of James I of England and the apothecaries of France despite a ban in favor of the Galenic remedies attempted by the Paris Faculté in 1603. It is no wonder that Paracelsus is still viewed as the father of medical chemistry.

Over time, as most of Paracelsus' formulae were adopted by mainstream academic medicine purely on a chemical basis, "the salt, sulphur, and mercury, which for Paracelsus were spiritual principles, operational definitions of physiological processes, became identified with these chemical substances as produced in the laboratory and were ultimately converted into the acids and alkalis. . . . Therapeutic practice was generated by chemical theory. Mechanics and hydraulics fulfilled similar functions."[23] And, of course, these medicines were administered solely on the basis of "opposites" in keeping with Galenic principles.

A full hundred years after Paracelsus, the Flemish physician Jan Baptista van Helmont developed a related version of alternative medicine. Like his predecessor, he gave priority to folk remedies, "for truly the Arabians, Greeks, or Gentiles, barbarians, wild country people, and Indians have observed their own simples more diligently than all the Europeans."[24]

More the scientist than the magician and visionary, Van Helmont explained disease as an idea or form imprinted on the vital force, or *Archeus* (in his terminology), which then "frames erroneous images to himself which should be unto him as it were for a poison . . . which images or likenesses, indeed, as being the seeds of disease beings, should be thenceforth wholly marriageable unto him in the innermost bride-bed of life."[25] Whether by direct reference to Van Helmont or in the general spirit of neo-Platonism, Hahnemann later suggested a vaguely similar mechanism for the implantation of pathological forms. The *Archeus*, though, may have a more exact match in the later theories of osteopaths and chiropractors, who propose energy and disease patterns transmitted from the spine, other bones, and cerebrospinal fluid to the viscera.

Medicines work not quantitatively against disease products (from Van Helmont's point of view, this was Galen's mistake in attacking the wrong source) but as specifics, unique wholes, from the ideas imprinted on their own *Archeus* which overcome the "idea" of the disease. Such "ideas" are scattered throughout creation and generate the character bases of individual people, the hidden morphologies of plants and animals, the rudiments of the various emotions, the invisible disease entities, and (happily) the seeds of medicines that can be manufactured from the effluvia of nature. This was a Renaissance variation on familiar Hippocratic, Celsan, and Paracelsan themes. It led to the homeopathic remedy typologies.

For reasons of holism Van Helmont generally opposed compounded medicines and other forms of polypharmacy. The disease is singular in relation to the organism and singular in what can cure it. "The sealing notes and impressions of diseases do not cohere with species," he wrote, "but with individuals only."[26] In general, Van Helmont retained the paradigm of nature as a vital entity, embracing a mysterious set of causes and effects, not subject to analysis, and operating only as a whole. He favored cure through coction, but it is interesting that, this far along in the history of the concept, it had been so totally confused with not only digestion but the assimilative and fermentative processes of each of the organs (which themselves had been clearly revealed through dissection) that Van Helmont himself could make no distinction between the vital force as a holistic entity and the individual mechanical functions of the body. It was not until Hahnemann that the complexity of this problem was even fully recognized.

More notably in terms of the mainstream thrust of medicine, the seventeenth century brought a new mode of scientific investigation (iatrochemistry) not dissimilar from Methodism and associated with Rene Descartes' view that if only enough experiments could be carried out, all motions in the universe and causes and their effects could be understood. Right up to Stephen Hawking and international chromosome mapping teams, we are still counting. Certainly, at that time, the discovery of the circulation of blood by the English physician William Harvey bolstered the mechanical metaphor. Harvey contributed his own interpretation: "The blood does not seem to differ in any respect from the soul or the life itself. . . . Nor is the blood to be styled the primigenial and principal portion of the body because the pulse has its commencement in it and through it; but also because animal heat originates in it, and the vital spirit is associated with it, and it constitutes the vital principle itself."[27]

Measurable geometry replaced ideal Platonic forms. Even life energy gained a geometric basis, hence did not require vital energy. Descartes wrote: "The food is digested in the stomach of this machine by the force of certain liquids which, gliding among the food particles, separate, shake, and heat them just as common water does the particles of quicklime, or *aqua fortis* those of metals."[28] The Cartesian Academy in France attempted to apply this theory to the Paracelsan theory of elements such that the characteristics of different salts were based on the shape of the corpuscles making them up (i.e., round for mobility and volatility, elongated and square for a fiery nature). It was not long before the actions of all drugs were explained by size, shape, and laws of motion.

A Dutch physician of the time, Hermann Boerhaave, wrote: "The solid parts of the human body are either membraneous pipes, or vessels including the fluids, or else instruments made up of these and more solid fibres, so formed and connected that each of them is capable of performing a particular action by the structure, whenever they shall be put in motion; we find some of them resemble pillars, props, cross-beams, fences, coverings, some like axes, wedges, levers, pullies; others like cords, presses, or bellows, and others again like sieves, strainers, pipes, conduits, and receivers; and the faculty of performing various motions by these instruments is called their functions; which are all performed by mechanical laws, and by them only are intelligible."[29] He rejected the notion of a vital force on the basis that "the material substrate cannot first accept the disease and then react against it unless permitted the attributes of autonomy and spontaneity."[30]

Empirical medicine was kept alive during the seventeenth century by a small number of others, including Giorgio Baglivi, an Armenian-born doctor raised and educated in Italy. Baglivi noted that the Galenists were not always successful in their cures, often evacuating bile without affecting fever and trying to heal too many conditions by focussing on acids and alkalis when "many diseases have nothing to do with acids and alkalis. Man has a thousand ways of being sick. . . ."[31]

The English doctor Thomas Sydenham complained that dissection merely showed the dead mechanism: "Though we cut into their inside, we see but the outside of things, and make but a new *superficies* for ourselves to stare at."[32] Sydenham shared a belief in the *physis* and the Law of Similars, i.e., that "fevers, evacuations, skin eruptions, etc., which occur in disease represent part of [the] healing effort." Fever is used by the *physis* "for the isolation of the tainted particles from the remainder of the blood."[33] Dysentery helps cleanse the intestines of morbific matter. Likewise, ulcers provide an escape route for harmful substances. The physician should assist vomiting and bleed women with suppressed menses.

In the early eighteenth century, one of the strongholds of Vitalistic medicine was the school at Montpellier, in France, that followed from the German Georg Ernst Stahl. Stahl was a chemist as well as a physician, yet he rejected pure chemistry on a humoral basis, and, in its place, he proposed that an intelligent force called *Anima* regulated the body. The circulation of the blood could be viewed not just as a hydraulic function but as the impulse of the *Anima* mediated through the nerves. It was by the movement of fluids that the *Anima* removed toxicities and kept the organism healthy.

Théophile Bordeu, a student at Montpellier, located his practice somewhere between Stahl and his *Anima* and the surgeons and physiologists of the medical establishment. Even as he upheld vital-force dynamics he tried to define them physically. The *Anima*, he said, regulated the flow of fluids through the body as a *chair coulante*, a circulating flesh, filling the pores and crevices, picking up extracts from the glands and carrying them to the organs. Bordeu wrote, ". . . a knowledge of the composition of the blood is inseparable from a calculation of the effects it produces unceasingly upon the sensitive organs."[34] Secretion is not a brute mechanical force; the *Anima* guides it intelligently and selectively through the organism. His research around such topics anointed him as one of the fathers of hormonal medicine, and he laid the groundwork for an understanding of the sympathetic nervous system and the involuntary responses of the body.

In line with the Hippocratic and Paracelsian traditions, Bordeu believed in curing by similars rather than contraries, and he revived the original principle of coction. Quelling the symptoms at crisis, he said, ensured only a continued history of chronic disease. He proposed that mineral springs were medicinal because they could transform chronic diseases into acute ones through inciting coction. He even dignified the cure-all theriaca, which was made up of all the leftover medicines from an apothecary's shop at the end of a day. Like the mineral waters, it was peppy and stimulative, capable of awaking the vital force from its languor or from its dwelling in melancholy and suppressed anger.

At this point, like theriaca, medicine was growing in creative chaos without a guiding principle. All of the notions and theories we have described (plus many others) had been floating around, interacting and subtly overlapping in every imaginable combination and set of tautologies and paradoxes for centuries, unresolved, drifting in and out of the mainstream. It was, at least, clear that Galenic, Cartesian, and iatrochemical medicine not only did not cure diseases consistently, but were singularly unsuccessful in instances of chronic disease. A new theory was needed to salvage a longstanding tradition of cure that had originated in the remote and unknown past, been partially catalogued in the original Hippocratic writings, and rediscovered and expanded by Paracelsus and the Paracelsan chemists. The later Empiricists were able only to patch around an expanding mechanist philosophy, borrowing its metaphors and occasionally losing their own meanings in ever-new simplifications of healing processes. Meanwhile, mechanism was taking over not only medicine but all of science.

Homeopathy is not the answer to all of these riddles, nor is it the sole destiny of either the Empiricist or Vitalist traditions of medicine. For one, it hardly speaks to much of Paracelsus' philosophy. It also does not address the original Eurasian elementalism that makes up the theory of humors. It does, however, represent what is perhaps the third major watershed of a mystery tradition—the first being Greek, the second being alchemical and neo-Platonic. Like the others, it is entirely unique and unexpected. Unlike the others, it has generated a cohesive and holistic theory that has moved throughout the world on its own and continues to ask its own homeopathic questions. Homeopathy was the single lucid offspring of all the shamanic chemistry, diagnosis by coction, search for quintessences and vital principles of substance that preceded it for centuries. In Hahnemann empirical medicine found its Galen.

Chapter 3

The Principles and Methodology of Homeopathic Medicine

1. DISEASES AND SYMPTOMS

Homeopathy differs from mainstream medicine on the most rudimentary level of definition, for it retains the Hippocratic tenet that the disease itself is unknowable. According to homeopathy, the diseases of standard medicine are classes of pathology representing not concrete illnesses but predispositions to weakness in the defense mechanisms of organisms. The diseases themselves are too profound, systemic, and spiritual for mankind to locate them. Dissections even of the living cannot reveal a disease or the curative process because they show only the flesh, and the flesh is animated in another plane. In his *Lectures on Homeopathic Philosophy*, published at the turn of the century, the American homeopath James Tyler Kent stated this fact in vintage homeopathic language:

> Causes exist in such subtle form that they cannot be seen by the eye. There is no disease that exists of which the cause is known to man by the eye or by the microscope. Causes are infinitely too fine to be observed by any instrument of precision. They are so immaterial that they correspond to and operate upon the interior of man, and they are ultimated in the body in the form of tissue changes that are recognized by the eye.[1]

The tissue changes are the visible result of disease on the inner plane. Any actual disease can generate a variety of widely different symptoms and symptom complexes in different individuals, none of which are the disease itself, none of which contain even a morsel of its actual fabric. Instead, these symptoms are the body's idio- syncratic response to the presence of disease. So much for the fabled disease armada of the Rationalists inherited more or less intact by modern medicine.

In homeopathic cybernetics, the organism is presumed always to generate the best possible (i.e., least destructive to itself) response to an underlying disturbance. It may develop painful and exotic pathologies, but even they will be the best it can manage under the circumstances. Its response is actually a system-wide recognition of the existence of disease within itself and a synchronous attempt to allow the disease (which is contemporary and inevitable) to express and vent itself with the least damage to vital organs.

If the best possible response is frustrated by medical treatment, then the organism will find the *next* best possible integration of the disease, i.e., the best possible response under the new situation. Although curtailment of symptoms might be considered cure by allopathic definitions, this is not the case in homeopathy. The dif- ference between the best possible response and the second best (or between any two sequential possibilities on this scale) may be the difference between eventual cure or lifelong chronic illness.

Ullman states these principles in contemporary language:

> For the past hundred years numerous leading physiologists and physicians have suggested that symptoms of illness do not sim- ply represent something wrong with the person, but rather that symptoms are adaptations of the body to stress or infection. Claude Bernard, the father of experimental physiology, acknowledged the impressive homeostatic tendency of the human organism.[2] Walter B. Cannon, author of the seminal book *The Wisdom of the Body*, rec- ognized the importance of the body's inherent intelligence.[3] Hans Selye, the father of modern stress theory, asserted, "Disease is not mere surrender to attack, but also the fight for health; unless there is a fight, there is no disease. Disease is not just suffering, but a fight to maintain the homeostatic balance of our tissues."[4]
>
> Systems theory lies at the basis of understanding symptoms as defenses. Systems theory assumes an interconnectedness of all things. It assumes that systems are intrinsically dynamic, that

equilibrium is stagnation and death, and that there are inherent self-organizing properties of a system once it achieves a certain level of complexity.

Different stresses upon a system cause it to adapt to that stress. An organism responds in at least two ways to a stress: it has general adaptive capabilities, and it also has the creative tendency to transcend previous defenses and develop new and potentially more effective means of reducing the pathogenicity of a stress. The system seeks to create a new level of order through fluctuation.

"Order through fluctuation" is a common description in physics of how systems adapt to change,[5] and yet, few scientists or physicians have considered that the body creates symptoms as a way that the organism seeks to create a new level of dynamic homeostasis.

From this perspective, therefore, a symptom does not necessarily represent the organism's collapse due to a stress or infection. Rather, a symptom is an adaptive reaction of the organism that represents the best possible response the organism can make based upon its present resources. It is, for instance, widely recognized that a cough is the body's efforts to clear the bronchials, that inflammation is the body's effort to wall off and burn out invading foreign bodies, that fever is the body's way to create an internal heated environment which is less conducive to bacterial or viral growth, and that the symptoms of a common cold are a response to viral infection, with the nasal discharge as the body's efforts to flush out dead viruses and dead white blood cells. Such are the body's impressive self-organizing, self-regulating, self-healing efforts.

With this understanding, the homeopathic law of similars is completely logical. Instead of suppressing symptoms, which then inhibits the organism's inherent defensive reaction, a homeopathic medicine is prescribed for its ability to mimic the symptoms of the sick person.

Just as the best way to control the skid of a car is to steer into the skid, perhaps the best way to heal ourselves of disease is to steer our body's own defenses into, rather than away from or against, symptoms. By aiding the body's efforts to adapt to stress or infection, the organism is best able to heal itself. Stewart Brand's description of homeopathy as "medical aikido" is thus perfectly apt.[6]

The conflict with allopathy is head-on here. If the visible disease is not the disease and if its alleviation is countertherapeutic, then the whole of medicine is involved in a system of superficial palliation leading to more serious disease. Doctors do not cure; they merely displace symptoms to ever less optimum channels of disease expression, each of which they (and insurance companies) consider to be a separate event because of its location in a new organ or region of the body. The disease meanwhile is driven deeper and deeper into the constitution because its preferred mode of expression is cut off each time.

As disease becomes more serious, it tends (by homeopathic interpretation) to change in the following manner: exterior organs improve, internal organs are affected in their place; symptoms move from the periphery of the body, typically the fingertips and toes, toward the center of the body, notably the heart and nerves; symptoms also move upward toward the head; life-sustaining systems are attacked last in the disease process; the acute becomes chronic with more severe and new acute phases in its cycle; temporary alteration of function becomes permanent alteration of structure; and pathology moves from the physical plane to the emotional plane to the mental plane, its ultimate expression being insanity and loss of reason.

The cure begins invisibly at the deepest level and works back out, symptom by symptom.

This is described eloquently by homeopath Edward Whitmont:

> No matter what the nature of the disturbance and the point of its appearance, it "wanders" through the whole organism from periphery to center, from less vital to more vital organs. A cure also operates in total-body fashion, but conversely, dissolving pathology in the opposite direction—from within outward, from the center to the periphery, from the more to the less vital parts. Demonstrating the non-local character of illness as well as the locus of healing, the cure moves also in the time dimension, re-evoking and subsequently abolishing symptoms and disorders in the reverse order in which the purportedly "separate" and "unconnected" disturbances originally occurred. The cure moves backward along the time scale, even over a whole life span. Former, less serious conditions that are thereby shown to have been earlier manifestations of the same, seemingly different disorder may temporarily return, only to be abolished automatically as the cure proceeds.[7]

On a simple physical level, homeopaths note sequences of worsening disease—for example: first herpes on the lips, then canker sores in the mouth, then canker sores deeper in the digestive tract, then duodenal ulcer, then colitis; or first a urinary infection, then a kidney infection, then cystitis, then nephritis, finally destruction of the kidney. These are single diseases, respectively, not different consecutive ailments.

A sequence indicating improvement could be, for example, severe heart attack followed by mild pneumonia (as the disease releases its hold on the heart and fans out into the lungs), then painful arthritis as it is dispersed to the joints. Its ultimate stage might be a return of childhood eczema. If the original condition was serious, the eczema itself may remain in mild chronic form for the patient's lifetime, a weakness grafted permanently onto the system. But certainly such a rash would be less debilitating than the other expressions.

It should be added that this kind of improvement, in the opinion of many homeopaths, can occur only from homeopathic medicines, though some admit the possible effectiveness of other dynamic medicines.

The disease, like the organism, vibrates through three hypothetical planes, which it integrates in its unity: the physical, the emotional, and the mental. In the spontaneous transfer of a disease from a more discrete material plane to a more organismic psychosomatic one, the new pathology must occur on roughly the same level as the old one, or a slightly worse level, but in shifting planes of manifestation, it can never improve. The shift itself is regarded as an inflammation. A skin ailment may appear to vanish without a trace, but the patient is suddenly depressed. A conventional doctor might wonder why. Shouldn't the patient at least be happy that the skin condition has cleared up? The homeopath knows why: the skin ailment was painful primarily because it expressed a deeper disorder. As the condition deteriorates and the disease itself comes closer to the core of the organism, it jumps to the emotional level and expresses itself as depression. The patient feels worse because he intuitively experiences the disorder closing in on him. The skin improvement is superficial. Conversely, the heart patient might well consider a rash to be minor and restorative after having felt the same disease in his heart. The skin ailment *is* the depression, or more properly, they are both functions of one aberration. Similarly, a stomach ulcer might be transformed into irritability or paranoia. It is the environment and defense system of the patient that determine how any condition will change and whether it will travel deeper on the same plane or be passed to a more interior one.

Chronic diseases never just "go away." That is too shallow and naive a prospect for the homeopath. A new pathology always replaces a disappearing old one. The old one may be presumed to be cured, but only because the organism's defense has retreated by a degree. This is how homeopathy salvages coction and the diagnostic art.

Standard medicine, in addressing visible pathology, must, by homeopathic rules, *always* drive disease deeper, for it deprives the organism of the best defense it has. But standard medicine will not recognize the translation; instead, the doctor will declare a cure or an alleviation. It is not that physicians are fools; any competent doctor understands the defense mechanism. Fevers, coughs, even ulcers are generally seen as healing responses, preventing more serious disease and useful except when they begin to cause organic damage themselves. Psychiatry also recognizes that the organism maintains the balance that best allows it to continue to function, and that without neurosis, the psyche would sink into deeper insanity or emotional fragmentation. Where standard medicine fails, by homeopathic standards, is in choosing a seemingly arbitrary point at which to break off its acknowledgment of defense priority and to begin an interventionist strategy. Allopathy, after all, believes that the skill of the physician can reverse certain conditions when the system cannot. Homeopathy proposes that systemic vitality alone can reverse pathology and that intervention on a symptomatic level must not only fail but do deeper damage by meddling with the organism's extraordinarily refined response.

In homeopathy, the visible disease is understood precisely as the symptomatic activation of the cure. The germs and microorganisms a disease attracts, the way in which it spreads and chemically alters the body—these in themselves are secondary to the dynamics of healing. Furthermore, temporary relief is always at the expense of a return to full health. From the point of view of homeopathic philosophy, symptomatic medicine is so widely accepted now in part because people do not know how true health actually feels.

The allopath is famously confused by temporary improvement because he does not view the organism as an entity with a single expression of disease. He never grasps the organized array of symptoms to see beneath them into the etiological relationship between events he considers isolated conditions. If, after allopathic treatment, a person with kidney disease has less albumin in his urine, the assumption usually is that the kidneys are working better. The patient may feel worse, but the doctor attributes that to a side effect of the disease, a matter for the psychiatrist, or an irrelevant concurrent happening. The homeopath treats nothing as a separate event. His experience warns that suppressed kidney disease may be followed by deeper discomfort, that the discomfort will not go away by itself, and that its cure will demand, on some level, the reexperiencing of the kidney symptoms. If that should actually happen, the original physician would consider it an unfortunate relapse. For the homeopath, though, it is the lucky reversal of suppression according to the therapeutic law that old suppressed pathologies represent themselves in reverse order when present ailments are correctly cured. This hierarchy is one of the keynotes of original Hahnemannian thought, as it was set down in the *Organon* (1810), Hahnemann's textbook of homeopathy:

> All diseases are, in fact, diseases of the whole organism: No external malady . . . can arise, persist, or even grow worse without . . . the cooperation of the whole organism, which must consequently be in a diseased state. It could not make its appearance at all without the consent of the whole of the rest of the health, and without the participation of the rest of the living whole (of the vital force that pervades all other sensitive and irritable parts of the organism); indeed, it is impossible to conceive its production without the instrumentality of the whole (deranged) life, so intimately are all parts of the organism connected together to form an invisible whole in sensations and functions.[8]

It is certainly clear from the above why a rapprochement between standard medicine and homeopathy is impossible. Just on the principles alone, without even including the exotic spiritual pharmacy, homeopathy condemns orthodox medical science to a wild goose chase of symptom classification that in no way reflects the dynamics of disease. In treating imaginary categories, physicians are doomed to mere guesswork, sophistry, or ultimate failure. Hahnemann wrote in the *Organon:*

> Two thousand years were wasted by physicians in endeavoring to discover the invisible internal changes that take place in the organism in diseases, and in searching for their proximate causes and *a priori* nature, because they imagined that they could not cure before they had attained to this *impossible* knowledge.[9]

Yet that "impossible knowledge" is the basis of all medical funding and research. It is what makes the National Institutes of Health, the March of Dimes, and Harvard Medical School legitimate organizations.

Homeopaths may sometimes reference the same physiology and biochemistry as their allopathic colleagues. But this knowledge is of little use in the treatment of disease, they feel, unless it helps link remedies to diseases or provides systemic-level clues. This is a devastating condemnation of medical practice. It is difficult enough for the average patient to accept that the doctor may have little understanding of or insight into the mechanism of their discomfort. But to allow that such information when attained—the pride of the establishment and twentieth-century enlightenment—is of no help in the actual treatment of disease is outrageous. Yet this is what homeopathy implicitly claims.

Modern homeopathy has developed a terminology to explain how conventional medical treatment must always make the patient sicker, even if it gives the passing illusion of health. Allopaths transform old well-known diseases into a new class of iatrogenic ailments that are difficult to unravel and often impossible to cure. If they prolong life in the process, they do so at a weaker level of vibration. George Vithoulkas, a contemporary Greek homeopath, explains these dynamics of false cure:

> Since allopathic drugs are never selected according to the Law of Similars, they inevitably superimpose upon the organism a new drug disease which then must be counteracted by the organism.

Furthermore, if the drug has been successful in removing symptoms on a peripheral level, the defense mechanism is then forced to re-establish a new state of equilibrium at a deeper level. In this way, the vibration rate of the organism is disturbed and weakened by two mechanisms: 1) by the influence of the drug itself, and 2) by interference with the best possible response of the defense mechanism. Consequently, if the drug is powerful enough, or if drug therapy is continued long enough, the organism may jump to a deeper level in its susceptibility to disease. The real tragedy of such a consequence is that the defense mechanism of the individual cannot then re-establish the original equilibrium on its own; even with homeopathic treatment of very high quality, it may take many years to return to the original level, much less to make any progress on the original ailment.

It is a strange but true paradox that people who have been weakened by allopathic drugging become relatively "protected" from certain infections and epidemics. This, of course, occurs because the center of gravity of susceptibility has moved so deeply into the more vital regions of the organism that there is not enough susceptibility on superficial levels to produce a symptomatic reaction. In such an instance, this is not a sign of improvement in health, but rather a sign of degeneration.[10]

So the successes of modern medicine may in fact represent anesthetization, systemic torpor, and deepening pathology.

Hahnemann offered the example of suppressed syphilis. First the external chancre is removed palliatively, the physician is satisfied, but the disease is deprived of its least dreary outlet. It may fester at the same level for several years, but eventually it will lodge more deeply, damaging the nervous system or the brain. Harris Coulter believes this precise process, over generations, has spawned AIDS.[11]

Take, for instance, the following sequence:

A sick person goes to a regular doctor. His or her disease is treated and he or she is considered cured.

The next time he (or she) is sick, he goes, perhaps unaware, to a homeopath who discovers that the new disease is primarily a result of the suppression of the earlier disease. Good therapeutics demands a return of that disease, which was ostensibly cured and the successful treatment of which was paid for.

By homeopathic standards, the patient is the victim of poor medical treatment. By allopathic standards, the patient was cured and came down with a new ailment. If he should return to the allopath, he would be told there is no invisible core disease and that the two separate physical diseases he has contracted are in fact different diseases. If he should return to the homeopath after that, he would learn that they are not different diseases, merely different symptoms of the same underlying disease. Ultimately a choice must be made. The allopathic establishment made that choice long ago, collectively, for the American public, but this does not do away with the problem. From a homeopathic point of view, the epidemic of allopathic medical care provided in civilized countries has driven disease inward to such a degree that we now see an exponential increase in the most serious pathological expressions—cancer, heart disease, mental illness, and immune-system deterioration.

Seventy years ago James Tyler Kent said that if we continue to treat skin disease palliatively, the human race will cease to exist. What a gargantuan exaggeration by the usual standards of medical theory! It is, in fact, inexplicable as stated. But homeopathy considers the skin a drain of bodily poisons and the first line of defense against diseases taking deeper root. If the outer layer reacts strongly, it protects the organism. Hence, skin disease is never trivial and should not be excised merely dermatologically.

The cumulative homeopathic charge of poor medical treatment against the doctors of the West is ultimately so serious as to be mind-boggling, and it places conventional malpractice in a totally new light. It is, finally, *all* malpractice. The difference, seen homeopathically, is between the sanctioned malpractice that makes up most of modern medicine and the occasional intentional or careless violation of a self-deceiving code of ethics.

The implications pyramid from here. If the disease is totally invisible, then most high-tech research is for naught. If medical treatment often provokes more serious ailments, for which patients must again be treated and charged, then the entire medical profession becomes an extortionist gang. The "sting" would outdo any con game on record. The older, sicker people, their diseases driven inward by earlier treatment, require extraordinarily expensive hospital treatment.

By this stage, the disease is so deeply internal that a full supporting army of laboratory, pharmaceutical, and surgical aid is required. The result can only be the death of the patient or the postponement of the jackpot until a later, even more serious and expensive ailment. Ultimately the patient dies, and the sting is complete, with legal disposal of the body. What makes the whole thing a mockery (again, we must emphasize, seen homeopathically) is that the *real* disease cause is invisible anyway. Any quest for its impossible object will become exponentially more expensive at each level of refinement, for as long as there is no limit to the variety and subtlety of equipment that can be developed to aid in this delusion, there is also no limit to the cost.

It is not that disease treatment has become more expensive with the improvement of techniques and the expansion of health care. It is that the medical profession has launched a Moon voyage-style expedition, with the public as unknowing guinea pigs *and* funders. While research has become ultraexpensive, actual health care has not improved on most fronts, except that of prolonging life. Unfortunately, the prolongation merely subjects people to more exotic or previously unknown diseases, with the result that they must continue to have their cases researched, though not cured.

The sick person is a participant in an ongoing lottery, allowed even to gamble on the results with insurance companies. He bets with his money that he will get sick and with his body and life that he will stay healthy. Either way, he wins, but either way, he loses.

An individual's control over his destiny, under this present medical regime, is limited to diet, exercise, and avoidance of certain obvious health hazards—all important and early Hahnemannian precepts anyway. But he may follow them to a tee and still get sick. Then he is subjected to medicines that may well prolong or deepen the illness. If he lives longer, it is in a devitalized condition, fodder for consumerist society.

Should there be any truth to these homeopathic views, here in our age of epic progress, when people are glad not to have been alive during times of plague, then we are somewhere else entirely, somewhere other than we thought we were. We would not be the first people in history to tread that ground. The age-old fear of

41

doctors that some people have may prove to be prophetic. It was once considered indulgent paranoia to fear the doctor, to believe that he somehow carried the illness and passed it on. Not by homeopathic standards!

This is the purest and most ideological version of homeopathy, one that is trapped in the nineteenth century and totally overlooks the progress of laboratory science, MRIs, CT scans and a knowledge of cellular and subcellular activities, to say nothing of atomic theory, fractals, and quantum mechanics. We now see so much tissue etiology that was recondite and inaccessible for millennia. To this degree homeopathy is dated science, though it reflects an important unexamined principle.

Symptomology *is* important in homeopathy, but it is used only diagnostically. Since the doctor is searching for a match to the disease among the remedies, he or she must learn to read symptom pictures. These are the sole basis on which to select a remedy. The disease cannot be assigned to a category and understood by characteristics common to the category. The disease is specific only to the one occasion of its appearance in the single patient, where, in delicate interaction with the defense mechanism, it leaves clues to its direction, hence the direction in which the proposed cure must work.

Coction is precisely and elegantly defined at last, after more than two thousand years of confusion. The disease is treated on the basis of the code of its symptoms, sparing the doctor any involvement in its ostensible nature or range of pathology. In Hahnemann's words:

> The disease, being but a peculiar condition, cannot speak, cannot tell its own story; the patient suffering from it can alone render an account of his disease by the various signs of his disordered health, the ailments he feels, the symptoms he can complain of, and by the alterations in him that are perceptible to the senses.[12]

The full import of this methodology may not come across in a first reading because we are accustomed to think of diseases followed by remediation. Our unconscious prejudice runs deeply enough for us to interpret homeopathic language only by allopathic clichés. But, since the true disease cause is unknowable, the cure *cannot* come from knowledge about pathology. The worst damage an ailment causes may tell us no more than any minor symptom, for both are expressions of a deeper-seated entity. Its ravages alone seem to require the doctor's exclusive attention (and well they should, for they may be life- or function-threatening); no wonder he endeavors to learn not only how such damage could come about but also how to reverse it.

Hahnemann, however, bypasses the whole matter of the relative importance of symptoms with a master stroke. All symptoms are important. The disease is a property of the constitution itself and lies beneath any concrete manifestation, beneath any separation into mental and physical. Everything potentially reflects it: a wart, a nightmare, a taste in food, a sensitivity to cold, diarrhea, weeping, anger, messiness, fastidiousness, fear, restlessness, loss of memory. Among symptoms recorded in a standard repertory (with the medicines of which they are descriptive) are: time passing too swiftly *(Cocculus);* crawling as of ants over the surface of the head *(Picric Acid);* calls his boots logs of wood *(Stramonium);* moved to tears welling at the sound of bells *(Antimonium Crudum);* symptoms worse at 2 A.M. *(Kali Bichromicum);* wounded pride *(Palladium);* feeling of a mouse running in the lower limbs *(Sepia);* feeling of a living animal in abdomen *(Thuja);* ridiculously solemn acts carried out in improper clothing *(Hyoscyamus Niger);* and a woman's dreaming of a large snake in her bed *(Lac Caninum).*[13]

Hahnemann knew that in a system of signs, unusual items carry more information than common ones. He writes: "In this search for a homeopathic specific remedy . . . the *more striking, singular, uncommon, and peculiar* characteristic signs and symptoms of the case of disease are chiefly and most solely to be kept in view."[14]

Odd as some of these symptoms may sound, each has a reason. The body wastes no energy. It would not be able to produce these morphologies unless it meant them (i.e., unless something inward spoke them). Hahnemann precedes Freud, the Structuralists, and the whole of twentieth-century humanistic and linguistic science in the dictum, "Either everything has meaning, or nothing has meaning,"[15] to paraphrase Claude Lévi-Strauss in *Totemism.* Freud tapped dreams, jokes, and compulsions as his clues to the unconscious; Lévi-Strauss later deconstructed ceremonies, kinship structure, and myths as the keys to the unknowable essence of a culture. Hahnemann used symptoms as pathways into the essence of a disease.

Hahnemann's insistence on replacing subjective value scales with precise record-keeping is decidedly modern. He understood implicitly that the evaluation of symptoms was a red herring that predisposed physicians into habitual disease categories. The only reason for emphasizing certain symptoms of a condition was to locate and name that condition in comparison with other conditions sharing those symptoms, then to treat it in a manner already set down as biomechanically effective for that pathology. But this was precisely the procedure homeopaths were to avoid.

Contradictorily, homeopathy gives the appearance, to the outsider, of being obsessed with trivial and odd symptoms. The homeopath tries to draw the patient out with a set of questions. He asks: "How do you feel before a storm?" "Do you close windows to prevent drafts?" "Do you find the house chilly or stuffy?" "Do you have times of more or less energy in the day?" "In what position do you like to sleep?" "How do you feel when your collar is buttoned?" "Do you like or dislike a belt around your waist?" "How do you tolerate waiting for a train?" He wants to know about degrees of jealousy and sadness, responses of frustration. He elicits fantasies and fears and dreams. He observes the patterns of rashes or pimples. He inquires into the color and thickness of urine and stools. He observes whether the patient is neat or sloppy. If he is neat, is he just neat, or fastidious? He may also ask "How do those around you think of you?"

A patient who recently suffered a heart attack may be astonished to find a homeopathic doctor more interested in his hand gestures while speaking, his ways of expressing anger, or a nightmare. If, in truth, homeopaths collected exotic symptoms because they believed each one needed to be improved, *sui generis*, homeopathy would be guilty of epic irrelevance.

This was never Hahnemann's intention. Homeopaths don't just collect and sort neutrally. They look for a striking symptom that unmistakably captures the whole—the constitution, the single character mask penetrating psyche and soma. The doctor elicits symptoms in order to find out the disease. Tastes in food hint at what the person is seeking or avoiding. Language describing sensations and tastes gives additional clues. Symptoms are the only visible remnants of an invisible attacker. If this intruder happens to track in a few grains of sand that show where he came from, the alert observer will use these and ignore the lamps he has knocked over and the bureau drawers he has pulled out.

The patient, especially when "trained" by allopathic symptom collection, will often ignore the most deep-seated and diagnosable symptoms and provide the ones that are most graphic and painful. But this is, of course, because allopathy does not make the same distinction between symptoms and diseases. When an allopath examines a diseased organ or a corpse, he is looking directly at proximate pathology. For a homeopath, these are only the hit-and-run effects of an assailant that has long since burrowed within.

Edward Tine writes, "Patients are so accustomed to their long sufferings, when the disease is chronic, that they pay little or no attention to the lesser symptoms which are often characteristic of the disease and decisive in regard to the choice of remedy. . . . Finally they leak out in some way and the patient says, 'I have always had it and did not suppose that it had anything to do with my disease.'"[16]

Esoteric homeopaths, as we shall see, believe that the true disease core is inherited. Hence, they elicit symptoms which appeared in childhood, even if they were once healed allopathically. Periodic acute conditions mark telltale outbreaks of an underlying disease in coordination with a defense response. The homeopath is interested in discovering the chronic sequence that incites in an acute susceptibility. But the patient may well have gotten so used to his long-standing problems that he discounts them and dismisses the possibility of improvement. No doctor has been interested in them before, so he forgets self-protectively and by habit.

As in psychiatry, when the verbal account of the symptoms is partly discounted as the patient's projection, the manner in which she or he gives information may itself yield the critical clues. The symptoms may then become less useful diagnostically than incidental office behavior. Many remedies (i.e., diseases) may be hypochondriac, talking about their ailments incessantly. *Nitric Acid*

45

is nihilistic as well, and will produce new, more dreaded symptoms if previous ones are relieved. It is a sterile anxiety with a conviction that no one can help under any condition. *Arsenicum Album* is just as anxious about his health, but he is convinced that the doctor can save him if only he will hear him out and get to the bottom of it. *Phosphorus* babbles about ill health, but not especially to the doctor and not with any sense that either his health or the doctor make a great deal of difference. *Tabacum* has a melancholic dread.

Hahnemann knew that a heart attack was more serious and worrisome than a wart or a craving for a particular food like broccoli, but as expressions of the constitution they are comparable. In fact, the craving for broccoli may suggest a medicine that the heart attack does not. The treatment by diagnosis from broccoli will then improve the heart condition in a way that emphasis on the immediate mechanical causes of the heart attack could not.

Put another way, the visible effects of pathology that stand out boldly and define the common disease groups of allopathy are often useless, for they define only the immediate acute phase. Cured alone, they may vanish, deepen, and return. Yet standard medicine not only emphasizes these but names its diseases after them and the classes they generate: tuberculosis, cancer, influenza, kidney stones, whooping cough, colitis, schizophrenia, acne, etc.

In homeopathy, diseases do not exist *at all* apart from their manifestation in individuals. "There are no diseases," wrote Hahnemann, in exact rendition of Hippocratic doctrine, "only sick people." A person has a singular constitution, although weakness in that constitution may be expressed differently at different times in his or her life. This is why a homeopath may claim to be able to cure one person's disease whose presenting complaint is a cancer, but after examining another person's skin rash may declare the disease incurable. To an allopath, this is a violation of fundamental reasonableness. But, homeopathically, names like "cancer" or "eczema" are simply shorthand for stages of totally different diseases that momentarily resemble each other in a stage of pathology, or that may have a transitory susceptibility to the same bacteria.

It is not biased to say that allopaths treat the *symptoms* of homeopathic disease—because allopaths do not believe there is a constitutional core. They consider the homeopathic inquiry a fantasy of vitalistic science; they are content to know the palpable disease. If homeopaths want to claim they can cure something more profound, allopaths leave them with the burden of proof that something more profound exists.

2. REMEDIES

The name of the homeopathic remedy is the name of the core disease; both generate the same symptoms. It is also, conveniently, the name of the patient's type. A patient treated with *Zincum Metallicum* has a *Zinc* disease (even if allopaths call it chicken pox, measles, eczema, or gastric diarrhea). Every pathological manifestation is *Zincum* at its roots. The constitutional type is likewise *Zinc*.

Zinc is sometimes recognized by complications in childhood diseases, eruptions which do not break out, with later neurological complications. *Zincum Metallicum* might also be recognized by bedwetting (especially when it occurs near morning), asthma (particularly in the evening) accompanied by farting, coughing in a reclining position, restlessness, and tics. In rare cases the clue to *Zinc* might be sleepwalking; the fact that severe diarrhea does not bother the patient; a dislike of wine, fish, veal, and sweets; or a dream of a horse that turns into a dog.[17]

Any of these rubrics may point to the remedy, or a combination of them may be determinative. For all intent and purposes the sum of them never occurs together. It is important to remember that the long lists of a remedy's attributes include *everything* known to be caused by a substance in every idiosyncratic individual; thus, they are always composites and exaggerations, even comically so. Only an unskilled homeopath looks for a match of the entire list or adds up corresponding items. A skillful homeopath looks for a distinctive symptom configuration that is congruent with a remedy, a sort of incomplete subset that could have no other source.

In general, disease cores (like chromosomes) send out messages which are expressed and suppressed at many different levels and which organize radically different tissue structures and states of being. The microdose is meant to correspond to the core, not to each peculiar expression.

Rhus Toxicodendron, a microdose prepared from an American Indian "herb," is distinguished by neuromuscular weakness approaching paralysis and by nutritional deficiency. It is also used when acute diseases progress in a typhoid direction into scarlet fever, diphtheria, dysentery, and pneumonia, as well as in cases of poison oak. A *Rhus Tox.* patient is often recognized by the fact that he or she is worse when resting, with the condition relieved by motion. Restlessness is a major diagnostic symptom. Other keynotes include joint pain (especially between 2 and 3 P.M.), a sore or dry tongue (sometimes coated but not at the tip), swelling of the eyelids, and a short ticklish cough originating behind the upper part of the sternum. *Rhus Tox.* is used for sprains and twists, and also for herpes, chicken pox, and shingles.[18] Because it resembles so many other remedies which share at least one of its major symptoms, *Rhus Tox.* must strictly be picked out not on the basis of single symptoms but by the relationships of elements in a symptom complex to one another.

Another herbal remedy, *Bryonia,* is prescribed for some of the same allopathically defined conditions as *Rhus Tox.* but differs in that it is worse from motion (even to the degree of having vertigo), is irritable and anxious, and experiences extreme thirst; its symptoms grow in severity from the mid-evening into the early morning (with 9 P.M. being a particularly bad time).[19] Hahnemann noted that upon "slight mental emotion (on laughing) there suddenly occurs a shooting (itching) burning all over the body as if he had been whipped with nettles or had nettlerash, though nothing is seen on the skin; this burning came on afterwards by merely thinking of it, or when he got heated."[20]

Tarentula Hispania, a spider poison, is recognized by crazed and tormented behavior—socially unacceptable deeds often regretted later. The patient is excited by music and sometimes perspires from melody or color. He or she sings and dances, has fits of nervous laughter, and masturbates frequently. There is pain and movement in the stomach and a sensation of insects boring and crawling on the limbs. Yet this remedy can be administered with barely any of the above symptoms in cases of constipation causing a person to roll from side to side or tumors around the vertebral column.[21]

Cocculus Indicus, an ancient fish poison, is indicated in some instances of extreme melancholy, deep reveries, difficulty concentrating, or speaking hastily (even wittily) without concern or sense. It is used also for vomiting, waking with a start from a hideous nightmare, and a number of cerebrally based disorders. It may be given for flatulent colic that is worse around midnight, especially in the context of an itching scrotum or early menstruation.[22] *Cocculus* has some of the same paralytic and anxious symptoms as *Rhus Tox.* and sings like *Tarentula;* thus, subtleties must be emphasized. Didier Grandgeorge notes *Cocculus* is often the remedy for people who attend to the dying and want to know the secrets of life. Such individuals may be naturally nosy and like to become doctors, nurses, and psychoanalysts.[23]

Nitric Acidum is usually an inflexible person who insists on following rules no matter what. If chastised, *Nitric Acid* will invariably make its own punishment worse. It is unforgiving of others. It loves fats and salt, especially herring. Physically, *Nitric Acid* includes chronic nasal discharges, otitis, white spots on nails, fetid perspiration of the feet, double vision, vertigo, and roaring in the ears. It is prescribed for brunettes rather than for blondes. People requiring it are chilly and depressed; they may have small, painful pimples on the tongue; and they find swallowing difficult because a morsel always sticks in the pharynx.[24]

Tine writes: "A patient comes with a pallid face, a rather sickly countenance, tired and weary, subject to headache, disorders of the bladder and disturbances of digestion, and in spite of all your questioning you fail to get anything that is peculiar. You prescribe *Sulphur, Lycopodium,* and a good many other remedies in vain. But one day she says, 'Doctor, it seems queer that my urine smells so strong, it smells like that of a horse.' Now at once you know that it is *Nitric Acid.*"[25]

Plumbum individuals are gloomy and depressed; they balk at constraints. They tend toward loss of memory, paralysis, sleeplessness, limb pain, stickiness in the throat, and numbness. *Lead* is distinguished by pale gums (sometimes with a blue line at their margin), blue swellings on the torso, lightning-like pains in the lower limbs and belly button (shooting to other areas), anemia and emaciation, the sensation in the throat of a ball rising into the brain, a disquiet that the abdomen and back are pressing together, an old-cheese smell to sweating feet, a hallucination that the feet are made of wood, urination drop by drop and scanty, and pain sometimes through to the bones.[26]

W. A. Boyson reports this *Plumbum* narrative from a patient: "'About six years ago I began to have crampy pains in my legs, sometimes twitching and burning and numbness. These pains were so bad that I could not sleep. For relief I'd get up out of bed, pound my legs, soak them in hot water, rub them with everything I heard of. I took a barrel of pills and gallons of liquids—no good. Finally I had a lumbar sympathectomy. That really was a mistake and I lost my sight for several weeks. The pain in my right toe became so severe that I had it amputated. Now my leg pains are worse than ever. How is that for a case?' 'Not bad,' quoth I, 'you have given me a beautiful picture.' A picture of what? Well, the five big remedies of central nervous system disorders are *Agaricus, Phosphorus, Plumbum, Picric Acid,* and *Zinc,* and this picture is that of *Plumbum.*"[27]

Pulsatilla, though it has physical manifestations such as circulatory problems aggravated by stuffy rooms, late menstruation, and frequent urging to stool followed by bellyache, is primarily a psychological remedy, at least in its repertorizing. *Pulsatilla* is often given to children, no matter their physical condition, who cling to teddy bears, suck their thumbs and, in general, have difficulty separating from their mothers. It is a remedy for disease caused by suppression of an early unhappy experience.[28]

Pulsatilla is an extremely emotional remedy, given to women whose lives are dominated by the people to whom they are devoted. A *Pulsatilla* person may be quite intelligent, but her emotions always trump her intellect. *Pulsatilla* is typically unsteady, moody, whimsical, and discontent; lachrymose, timid, and phlegmatic. *Pulsatillas* are said to favor old-fashioned blouses and the color blue. They are often blonde with blue or green eyes and round faces. Many of them sweat on only one side of their bodies and/or are almost superhumanly thirstless. They hate fatty foods but love butter to the point of craving. Their pains wander, with rheumatism going from joint to joint. They may sneeze a lot, chatter in their sleep, and, though feeling chilly, find external heat intolerable. They tend toward hypochondria with great enough anxiety to want to throw off all their clothes.[29]

Finding the essence of *Pulsatilla* can be difficult. It closely resembles *Silica, Phosphorus, Lycopodium, Calcarea,* and a number of other remedies. Hahnemann lists 1156 separate symptoms. Later provings have brought the number up to close to two thousand.[30]

Tuberculinum is made from a potentized disease product, tuberculous lymph nodes. In fact, many of the early homeopaths considered it so loathsome they resisted using it. Now it is a standard part of the repertory, especially for dealing with the tubercular aspects of miasmatic disease layers.[31]

Tuberculinum is fundamentally restless but not in an aimless way; he longs to be free of whatever he is doing or wherever he is, experiencing a constant desire for travel (to the point of globetrotting), consciousness-expanding drugs, and sometimes competitive and physical sports. This is a highly intellectual type who craves new stimulation and, while being naturally curious, often lacks depth of inquiry, mental patience, or the ability to sustain any one quest. Because of his hyperactivity, *Tuberculinum* keeps changing the subject of his attention. Another indication of this type is that no other remedy works for any length of time, and many seemingly correct remedies have only temporary effect. *Tuberculinum* is (by approximately five to one) a male remedy.[32]

Tuberculinum is susceptible to allergies, deathly afraid of animals (especially dogs), has acne as a teenager, and is improved from staying in the mountains (but not above 5,000 feet, which is too arousing for him). He loves open air or riding in a brisk wind and tends to open windows everywhere, but afterwards he is susceptible to persistent colds and catarrhs. The *Tuberculinum* individual tends toward headaches and / or constipation followed by diarrhea during which he suffers heavy sweating. *Tuberculinum* can also be emaciated, "thin as a rail," and hypersensitive to changes in the weather.[33]

People needing *Tuberculinum* as a remedy often have tuberculosis in their family and receive the BCG (tuberculosis) vaccine without effect. The vaccination causes swollen glands; its scar gives off pus. However, *Tuberculinum* is not just a cure for tuberculosis or tubercular miasms; it is a distinct character type of its own, of which tuberculosis is but one of many possible manifestations.[34]

3. SIMILARS AND REMEDY RESPONSES

Since the organism's own defense mechanism is already the first remedy, the homeopathic medicine should be an amplification or support of its work. By the Law of Similars a patient is given a remedy that would produce symptoms similar to his disease in a healthy person, and thus can respond directly to the medicine itself. A successful cure matches a medicine's often toxic and emotionally disturbing effect with a disease pathology. If the doctor does not know such a medicine from experience, she must find candidates in the Homeopathic Repertory, which is essentially the collected history of two centuries of individuals' responses to remedies. Many medicines will partially mimic the disease. After narrowing her choice down to a few, she must choose the Similimum, the specific remedy, on the basis of her comprehension of the wholeness of the disease and the matching wholeness of the remedy. Although individual symptoms and characteristics are useful in finding one's way through thousands of possible remedies, ultimately the doctor must deal with the fact that remedies and the diseases to which they correspond are functional wholes and express characteristics and tendencies that go beyond a simple multiplicity of symptoms. In practice, homeopathic diagnosis falls somewhere between an encyclopedic research project and an instantaneous comprehension of a unity.

Again, we must remember homeopaths are trying to cure symptoms by trapping their whole underlying disease and thus catching them up efficiently and miraculously in one net. The medicines have no virtue and no rationale beyond their fortuitous mirroring of a disease. That mirroring alone makes them curative.

The only practical information about remedies thus comes from their testings and uses. Disease and medicine are matched without insight into the mechanism of the former or the chemistry of the latter. It is Hahnemann's first law of homeopathic pharmacy "that it is only in virtue of their power to make the healthy human being ill that medicines can cure morbid states, and, indeed, only such morbid states as are composed of symptoms which the drug to be selected for them can itself produce in similarity on the healthy."[35]

Another way to look at homeopathic treatment is to posit that ideally, the disease itself could be the medicine, but for deep-seated reasons of constitutional inertia, environmental toxicity, social disruption, genetic weakness, whatever, this is no longer (if ever it was) the case. While an organism is always able to improve within certain symptomatic limits, it cannot spontaneously throw off an entire illness that matches its own basic susceptibility, so it will succumb in time. For one, the illness exists in layers, without a single shape or dynamism, so it can insinuate itself. A correct remedy then allies with the defense mechanism and jars the system out of the disease configuration. Many additional remedies may be needed after the first one before the full archaeology of the condition is dislodged.

Actually, past conditions cannot be treated unless a removal of present symptoms brings them back. Hence, chronic ailments that are in temporary dormancy cannot be diagnosed and engaged until they actually recur. The mirror of the Similar ripples and re-forms differently.

Each remedy, as it is given, changes the picture. It is briefly the single remedy, but as soon as the picture changes, another single remedy replaces it. Ultimately, a series of these "single" remedies will unravel and dispel the entire condition. It is crucial that they be administered only one at a time, for no grand singular cleansing is possible. Each new picture is interpreted only in terms of its priority and the response of the system to the last remedy given.

Jonathan Shore, who is both a homeopath and an M.D., notes: "After taking a remedy it is important to watch closely for changes. Remedies may begin their action by an improvement in the emotional area, by an aggravation of symptoms, by a general improvement, or other more subtle responses . . . Sometimes a good response is a small change in some insignificant-seeming symptoms that show us indications for the next remedy."[36]

By the standard of an eventual, complete cure, a symptomatic alleviation is not as important as successive pictures, for as long as the present picture is clear, a more correct remedy can always follow a less correct one—a more accurate Similar. The only incorrect choice is a remedy that clouds the picture and confuses the sequence of prescriptions.

This does not mean that functionally homeopaths do not hit a working remedy on the first try. They do. My version is a collective idealization of a complete cure, something rarely attempted. In the ideal case, of which actual cases are abridgments, the levels of disease must be separated, one by one, as the physician goes, etiologically, from one whole picture to the next whole picture. He cannot predict what will appear next, and he must not be dismayed if a new condition brings more pain or disability than a previous one. Homeopathy is nonpalliative by principle. It often causes suffering, unwinding a disease by a passage through the elements that make it up in time and space. A successful sequence may pass through painful eruptions, especially if the disease is deep-seated and has been suppressed by antibiotics or steroids. Superficially, things get worse. However, if the flare-ups did not occur, the entire disease could not be located and healed. The process might stalemate around a particular pathological equilibrium, symptom-free but apathetic.

One does not know, before the fact, what will happen, for the process unleashes its own dynamics, its own history, as it goes. The basic homeopathic law applies at each new level: prescribe by similars; take a total symptom picture and administer the remedy that would cause those symptoms; wait while the organism fights for a new equilibrium; and when the result of the treatment is finalized, take a new picture; prescribe again if necessary.

Each prescription assumes that the organism will cybernetically make the best possible use of the dose, even if it is not on exactly the wavelength of the disease, and that the results of the prescription and subsequent reorganization then will define the next phase. The patient is improved only if he is organized around a less inward and profound center of gravity of disease. If he is reorganized around a deeper center of gravity, the medicine has made the condition worse. If the medicine is totally off the wavelength of the disease, then nothing will happen and the doctor will have a fresh chance. A very errant prescription does not alter the case at all, whereas a near-miss may cause a disruption which, if it is not antidoted, will make the disease worse, the picture muddier, or both.

Each condition, as it comes into being, is real. It does no good to say: "That *was* the disease. Let's refer back to it." It is no longer *the* disease after the remedy.

The lay physician Theodore Enslin, in a seminar in 1977, described how, when the symptoms drop off, they go back in time:

> In the treatment of a condition, a conditioning which has gone on for many years, sometimes it is not possible to cure with one shot; it's not a miracle at all. That's one reason a good prescriber wants to know as much about the patient as possible: everything. So you begin a reverse process. You begin, very practically, with what is exactly there. When those symptoms are cleared, very often you will find that that patient has symptoms that are prior, of things that happened before that. And you keep on going. You go back to childhood. And there are many stories about the actual walking off of the last symptom. You get to the point where it will go right off a finger, the last wart or pain. There are many case histories like that. Sometimes this process can take a number of years.[37]

The keynote of practical homeopathy is the correct interpretation of sequential pictures from the administration of remedies. Kent, for instance, gives twelve very careful "observations" to make after the medicine is given:[38]

The first is that when there is prolonged aggravation of the symptoms, followed by the final decline of the patient, it means too strong a medicine: the action was too deep for the degree of deterioration that had already taken place, and the weakened vital force was unable to throw off the new attack. Since the medicine can work only through the vital force, the physician must assess how strong the vital force is before giving a remedy. The potency of the medicine must be harmonized, approximately, to the capability of the vital force.

In the second observation, there is also a long aggravation, but one leading to slow and final improvement of the patient. In this case, the disease was deep but deterioration was not as great, hence the medicine was appropriate. The aggravation was long because tissue change had already taken place.

The third observation is that if there is a quick strong aggravation, followed by rapid improvement, the remedy was correct, and no serious tissue change has taken place.

In the fourth observation, where there is recovery without aggravation, Kent wonders if there was any disease in the first place or if the disease was relatively new and superficial.

In the fifth observation, improvement and amelioration of the symptoms followed by aggravation indicate that the disease is deeper than the medicine and the medicine was acting only palliatively.

The sixth observation is slightly different: short relief followed by return of the symptoms might mean the patient has antidoted the remedy by coming into contact with substances that neutralize the potentization.

In the seventh observation, the symptoms are relieved, but the patient still feels sick. This means the wrong medicine because there are latent organic conditions preventing a cure.

In the eighth, the patient proves every remedy. This may be an idiosyncrasy; it may also indicate an incurable condition. Kent suggests using a higher potency.

The method of bringing on symptoms in a healthy person by giving a medicine is known as proving (the ninth). It is a procedure for discovering new remedies and is considered beneficial in an immune-stimulating way to people who do it.

New symptoms might also indicate a proving, which would mean the wrong medicine had been used (the tenth). It is important, however, to distinguish between a proving and the reappearance of old symptoms. When old symptoms reappear in the reverse order of their original occurrence (the eleventh observation), this confirms that the healing process is moving in the natural direction.

In the twelfth observation, the symptoms move from without to within, driving the disease deeper. This indicates the doctor prescribed only for a peripheral condition, and in so doing hastened the disease process.

Looking beneath the surface of such indications, Whitmont emphasizes the nondichotomizing aspect of the application of single holistic doses in all energy medicines:

> There is no malefic-beneficial dualism: toxic or potentially damaging agencies may also serve genuine healing when applied with due regard to organismic integrity. The needle in the hand of the acupuncturist, the knife in the hand of the surgeon, microdoses of arsenic administered according to the homeopathic simile principle all may heal when used as a means of harmonizing, balancing and reintegrating overall psychosomatic functioning. When aimed at isolated functions, however, they serve to forcibly change one part, hence evoking a compensatory imbalance of others. Then such remedies become irremediable.[39]

By esoteric homeopathy, the same diagnosis applies to the collective health of humanity. Our supposed global improvement of health and longevity betrays on deeper levels what it conceals by its propaganda. We might say that some isolated conditions are better (smallpox and polio, for instance), while others are worse (like cancer, mental disease, immune deficiencies, genocide), but that would violate holism, and from a homeopathic standpoint, social and economic problems are deemed the collective result of disease driven inward. So smallpox may turn into sociopathic behavior over generations of suppression masking as cure. A palliative reduction of tuberculosis can lead to an increase in criminal activity. Harris Coulter addresses this problem in his famous book on the relationship between vaccination and social violence.[40]

The same solution is applied to the planet as to any individual: its case must be taken now, and the prescription must address present symptoms. Only when these are changed can a new prescription be given. There is no way to return now to the times of simpler diseases and apply homeopathic remedies on that basis.

In an ostensibly healthy person, the effects of the homeopathic remedy are manifested as a brief artificial disease called a "proving," because it is the only proof of how the medicine will behave in a sick person. The initial contribution of a homeopathic remedy is to aggravate the disease, while the initial effect of an allopathic drug is to alleviate the symptoms. However, it is not the initial effect of the medicine that is of concern homeopathically. The homeopathic aggravation must be followed by swift and deep cure in the case of the correct remedy. The allopathic alleviation is palliative and insubstantial; it drugs the organs without strengthening their response. The only lasting effect of an allopathic pharmaceutical on the system is its side effect, which is chronically and ultimately aggravating. This, of course, does not banish allopathic drugs as shams, but it does mean they should be used solely in a conscious attempt to stop serious infections, remove carcinomas and dangerous growths, free arteries, etc. Then, when the patient is safe, a deeper and more holistic treatment can occur.

When a homeopathic aggravation occurs in a sick person, this is, in a sense, the result of an artificial disease and an actual disease combining before the dynamics of that fusion provoke a new condition. The aggravation is not always even noticed. Since the condition may already be painful and intense, and since the vibration of the medicine may well occur on a deep organic level, its shock may blur with one's general kinesthesia. Contrarily, if the person has been under suppressive allopathic treatment which has been halted for the substitution of homeopathy, the aggravation may be more painful than the disease, for it will activate something that had previously been drugged and to which the organism had been artificially numbed.

If the remedy is right, though, patients always sense they are better. Every obvious manifestation may be worse, but there is an intuition that things are under control and will improve, a feeling of well-being.

The question then is: Why is the homeopathic remedy so much more noticeable to the organism than everything else in the environment? Homeopaths give two answers: 1) it is exactly specific, and 2) it is on the dynamic plane.

Because the disease always is the precisely correct response of the defense mechanism to an overall condition, the organism engages with it, as it were, in a folly, even to the death. The medicine resembles the illness, often to a tee, but it is *not* the illness, so it fools both the organism and the disease. The vibration of the matching remedy provides a safe context, somewhere in the internal language of the body, for the expression of a pathological predisposition. The deeper sickness is relieved by the Similar, the "nonpathology," instead of by a deteriorative disease.

That is one model. But we might also say the medicine generates psychophysically and morphogenetically what was *constitutionally* lacking so that a deficiency is not expressed pathologically. Perhaps also the medicine shocks the system into action, causing it to cure itself. Enslin said:

> It is a parallel. It is a recognition of the fact that the unwanted manifestations can only be braked by producing other unwanted manifestations which are similar. And there's a great difference between similar and the same. There's a popular conception: if the guy gets gas from eating cabbage, you give him a high dilution of cabbage, and that's going to cure him. That's not what's done at all. Actually, the medicines are not medicines at all. The process is an outrage of the system itself. A diseased system is an apathetic one: it just doesn't give a damn. But in many—most cases, unless the thing has gone too far—that apathy can be overcome by introducing a parallel. When that parallel becomes apparent to the organism, it's outraged—and cures itself. The medicine actually has very little to do with it.[41]

Homeopaths understand that it is ultimately the vital force that cures, not the medicine. Disease is a force of nature, like gravity or procreation. To assume that it could be manipulated by crude machines or concoctions of physicians is arrogant. One might as well, with Ahab, attack the Sun. The only rival to the disease is the life essence of the organism. If that can be sparked into countering the disease, then even the most severe ailment can be overcome. A nonhomeopathic use of crude substance or mechanism to alter its course, however, must end up being as much an attack upon the organism as it is upon the disease.

Hahnemann scoffed at the idea that a medicine could be instructed to do only good when in the body. One might as well, he wrote, instruct the carbon, nitrogen, and hydrogen in a meal of cabbage, roast beef, and wheatcakes, telling them what part of the body to nourish and what part to stay out of. Yet this has been pretty much the only game in town. His escape from such a dilemma was to substitute nonmedicines for medicines, i.e., substances which affected the system not by digestion or assimilation but by the nonlinear information they carried to the cellular and subcellular levels of tissue. Then the native intelligence of the body and the disease, matched in the insight of the physician, might fuse in a cure.

Whitmont takes us right to the heart of the paradox:

> In terms of our accustomed understanding of biology and physiology, it seems incredible that spasms are relieved by a dose of "no-thingness," and "absence" of something that in its material form would cause spasms. What of the corollary fact that when we further attenuate this "no-thingness" it becomes more intensely effective? How are we to understand that a "non-existent" dose of Spanish fly, a blistering and abortive agent in its material form, does away with the effects of second-degree burns and can even be life-saving and infection- and shock-protective in third-degree burns, and that it exerts this effect not from local application but after ingestion orally? How can we explain that a dematerialized potency of ordinary table salt, a substance we consume daily, regardless of this daily consumption, can alleviate sorrow and grief and their somatic effects as well? Or that Arnica, a plant growing on high mountain meadows, protects against the effects of mountaineering accidents and contusions, sprains, concussions, and physical but also emotional shock?
>
> Homeopathy provides a virtually paradigmatic instance of the phenomenon of inner-outer correspondence by non-material information which has been simultaneously recognized and ignored throughout human history. We find this phenomenon in African drumming rituals, Navajo sand-painting ceremonies, Tibetan visualization techniques, as well as various systems of healing by mantra and faith, Japanese Reiki, the polarity therapy developed by Randolph Stone in India, and even apparently concrete treatments such as hydrotherapy, herbal baths, aromatherapy and skeletal manipulation.[42]

A system like homeopathy cannot in fact work as substance. It is a medicine of the shadow of technology. Its validity—its capacity to heal—comes at least in part from its denial of the overendowed material and junk flooding the modern world, i.e., its defiance of biochemical priority. I would imagine that a medicine of "nothing"—which is, by the way, what the AMA considers homeopathy—has unique potential in an age clogged with overproduction, vapid data, and quick-acting palliatives. Homeopathy tells us that the whole commodity bureaucracy is "nothing" also, the life it endows is "nothing" as well. It (and the other energy medicines) carry the full power of the uncompensated-for spirit—the Aboriginal drum—inside us. They are allopathy's true enantiodromia. In fact, they are our only present clue to what may be a whole nether universe of matter and energy—a realm shrouded in darkness and obscurity and a conspiracy of silence in our time.

4. MIASMS

In esoteric homeopathy, diseases are layers, patterns imposed upon each other. The disease of any one person is built up of historically successive miasms. These miasms, at any given moment, describe a totality; since the organism is a unity, they are a unity. In the classic model the doctor must begin by prescribing for the current miasmatic layer, as he perceives it, ignoring temporarily any deeper levels contained within it. If he removes the outer miasmatic level, the pattern will oscillate, presenting a new picture.

The number of prescriptions necessary is determined by the miasmatic depth of the disease, which is not at all the same as its intensity or pathology. These may well be minimal in a deep miasmatic disease because then the defense mechanism is not strong enough to produce a vibrant response. Systemic apathy is too great. Likewise, an intense disease does not mean a deep miasmatic condition. It could indicate a healthy defense system, except in the final throes of long chronic disease before ultimate demise.

Acute disease is then nothing more than a stimulation of the defense mechanism by a pathogenic agent. Chronic conditions likewise incorporate agents to which they are responsive in order to provoke eruptions with the ultimate aim of getting better. In homeopathic epidemiology pathogenic bacteria, far from being freelance invaders, increase and decrease in the organism only according to the disease level and its requirements. Very contagious ailments (i.e., agents) affect large numbers of contiguous people, but, even so, not all people and not all people in the same way. It is the defense mechanism and intrinsic disease level that always determine the nature and expression of the response to environmental entities. The morbific agents, on which standard medicine focuses in its interest in common symptoms and categories of cases, are secondary to the individual responses of organisms. Each organism will use the occasion of the "bug" to express its particular chronic needs. Thus, each organism still requires individual treatment even in an epidemic.

Sometimes a morbific agent itself is so severe as to be life-threatening. It may be powerful enough to impose consistent symptomology on a large number of people. In such pandemic circumstances, homeopaths may well use a limited repertoire of remedies or even a single remedy for all people. That is an admission that the disease itself is too powerful a "medicine" at this stage of history for people in our society to individualize. It is like a vast, generalized poison, or germ warfare. But there are no absolute values with regard to disease. An epidemic is potentially exteriorizing, hence cleansing (like coction), but its manifestations are life-threatening and, if they are not alleviated, the organism will not survive. A homeopath may agree to antidote this challenge of nature (in the form of an overly toxic "medicine") with an allopathic drug, recognizing that the person is not ready to handle such strong cleansing. Treatment may fail, and the patient may be lost. Homeopaths can no more cure all conditions by Similars than they can negate death. They can only engage the organism in the most creative and curative response of which it is capable. The universe meanwhile will continue to generate new challenges along the path of evolution.

A homeopath uses allopathic pharmacy to antidote. He can impose an allopathic drug to antidote a bad homeopathic prescription, he can also use one to "antidote" a life-threatening disease which is natural miasmatic medicine. From an esoteric homeopathic standpoint, homeopathy is a creative use of artificial diseases to bring about human transformation and, ultimately, health; allopathy is a means of antidoting dangerous but creative disease processes. Real homeopathy is in a sense the invisible curative cycle of the biosphere working at a mysterious quantum level throughout the planet (and cosmos) without even the crude invention of homeopathy-like medicine. It is required now—and has come into being— only because the human race has fallen out of balance with the invisible "homeopathic" processes of nature. Organisms in harmony with their environment generate or find their own homeopathic cures outside the context of formal medicine.

Homeopathic philosophy understands society, the environment, and organisms as being in counterbalance with a process of vitality and disease. A morbific agent arises when the overall civilizational process requires it at some level. If individuals die, it is as they die in nature: the disease itself is not their death knell—it is ironically their opportunity, their civilizational opportunity, to escape a particular stagnation through the deepest possible realignment. That is, disease is like a harsh Zen master demanding change at a core level and dealing out pain and death when that change does not occur. This is a shamanic ceremony that never ends.

All other political and economic solutions are palliatives, doomed attempts to make the law of contraries work.

For instance, the present ecological crisis of the West is a plague of symptoms. If humanity were transformed (and disease is surely its intrinsic, inevitable, transforming agent), then solutions would emerge from within the crisis. In that sense, the disease level of the world is an elegant systemic response to all its problems. Likewise, pollution incites our collective immune response.

From a Hahnemannian standpoint, slaughter in Somalia or Cambodia or Guatemala is the work of miasms driven inward to the mental plane and on an epidemic level. Pornography, sexual violence, ghetto riots, mayhem in the United States, and terrorism and ethnic cleansing in Europe are diseases, attempts to resolve imbalances in the only way the organisms themselves know how. The murderer-rapist so little understands his deed because he *is* his deed. In his acts of torture and erotic cannibalism Jeffrey Dahmer was sicker than a victim of AIDS because his system was unable to galvanize a physical disease response. He was truly apathetic, degenerate.

Despite the horror it provokes in us, we almost expect such depravity and would be disappointed without it. We would be disappointed because we know that we can't ultimately recover and survive otherwise. Unconsciously we hope our sensitivity is still great enough to respond with pathology. In this way, carrying out the madness of the Vietnam war relieved the United States of the premonition of a far deeper disturbance that was long brewing. The innermost layer erupted into pathology. People intuitively understood that we were collectively sicker before the disease, though we looked calm and happy during the preceding decade.

Allopathy deals with society as it deals with the body: experiences of life are considered separate and unconnected; roles are temporary and circumstantial. An ailment of the liver is an ailment of the liver, and a job driving a bus is a job driving a bus. If a bus driver has a liver malfunction and cannot go to work, the allopath attempts to return him to work. His liver is "improved," and he can drive the bus. He can re-inhabit his job, his family, his general social station.

Homeopathic treatment tries to change the entire organism. Jobs and social situations may be part of the disease; thus, when patients start to get better, they may find themselves unable to fill the same roles in society. When they continue in old paths, their illnesses may return. The larger treatment requires an adjustment of all circumstances, organic and environmental, in which the patient finds himself. The liver ailment and driving the bus are no longer interdependent circumstances, but different layers of *the same thing.*

The deepest individual disease is genetic and congenital; an organism inherits the constitutional predispositions and weaknesses of its ancestors and even its species. Onto the genetic level are imposed the miasms of early childhood diseases and conditions suppressed by allopathic medicine or otherwise internalized. Onto this level are imposed a series of chronic and acute diseases and allergies (the latter of which are simply the heightening sensitivities of the chronic to external aggravation), and then the exact environmental conditions to which the organism is exposed, including the social order, the economic system, the spiritual stage of the society, and chemical pollution. These different webs may be integrated in a variety of ways, but the patient is a dynamic expression of all the forces that penetrate him, which have brought him or her into being and which sustain his or her world.

In esoteric homeopathy, the deepest cure must always be sought, initially at the risk of the patient's balance, job, and relationships, and ultimately at the risk of his life. At the same time, the physician no doubt realizes that absolute cure is an impossibility because the disease is in civilization.

Practical homeopathy compromises on the level to which it will seek cure. The physician may decide not to treat a certain depth of an ailment if he feels that the patient has no space into which to expand and make room for the cure, or if he can live a decent, healthy life without such a cure. If diseases and life situations are in a state of balance, any one disorder may be part of a necessary homeostasis for the survival of the patient. A strong remedy can have suicidal consequences if the patient cannot integrate the new implications. It is also possible that a mental remedy can be driven back onto the physical plane in a debilitating or life-threatening way. One homeopath reported treating a patient who had been chronically ill until she joined a very expressive religious sect. She felt better but became fanatic and unhappy. Soon after taking a remedy, she lost interest in religion and developed multiple sclerosis. Perhaps, the doctor argued, the ailment returned to its new corresponding point on the physical plane, protecting the mental plane.

Many doctors who use homeopathic remedies dismiss this entire esoteric interpretation of disease and human history. They practice by habit not theory. They do not know how people get sick or why certain methods cure them, or even if these methods are the causes of the cures. Any candid discussion with the allopathic family doctor reveals similar mysteries at the heart of all successful treatments.

However, the lapses of conventional medicine are covered by familiar jargon. Its enigmas have been integrated into our social expectations and cultural superstitions in a way that allows everyday discussion of ailments and cures without deeper understanding, even as the costs of an often tautological system of diagnosis and treatment skyrocket. The allopathic disease names are still the common names for diseases, and as taxonomic entities, they become half of the explanation and half of the cure.

5. MICRODOSES AND THE VITAL FORCE

The vital force is the seed of life. Since it is unitary as well as primal, it ensures the singleness of the disease and the single effect of the medicine. Disease is a distortion of the vital chord that is transferred to the physical body as susceptibility. When the precisely correct medicine (the Similimum) hits the body at any point, the vital force uniquely recognizes it. Homeopathic theory does not confer the power of dynamic readjustment on medicines or the organs themselves, only on the vital force. Hahnemann writes:

> This *dynamic* action of medicines, like the vitality itself by means of which it is reflected upon the organism, is almost purely *spiritual* in its nature. . . . This dynamic property is so pervading that it is quite immaterial what sensitive part of the body is touched by the medicine in order to develop its whole action . . . immaterial whether the dissolved medicine enter the stomach or merely remain in the mouth, or be applied to a wound or other part deprived of skin.[43]

It is certainly immaterial when it is projected psychically, as it is by some homeopathic healers!
Whitmont notes:

> A homeopathic potency once produced lasts indefinitely and can always be perpetuated without any loss in intensity by simply adding new solvent. Nor can psychic induction be quantified or shown to be subject to entropy. Einstein's formula $E = m/c^2$ does not apply, there being no masses, energies or velocities.[44]

Homeopathic medicines are "spiritual" medicines. Despite their elaborate chemical preparation by an overt laboratory procedure, they are not drugs (though legally they are over-the-counter drugs). The final product, the actual pill, is such a high dilution of the original substance that nothing is left of it; in some cases, an infinitesimally tiny amount, not known to have any biomechanical effectiveness, remains incidentally. The actual procedure is as follows:

The medicinal substance, which might be plant tincture, animal product, mineral, disease discharge, or, in fact, anything that one chooses, is diluted in nine parts neutral medium. If it is a liquid or soluble in alcohol, then alcohol is used and the new solution is shaken vigorously after dilution. If it is not soluble in alcohol, then it is pulverized (triturated) in a mortar with milk sugar. This operation is used for silica, animal charcoal, graphite, sulphur, crude antimony, gold, platinum, zinc, copper, silver, tin, a variety of carbonates, and other alcohol-insoluble materials. The process, carefully defined by Hahnemann as to the amount of milk sugar and the technique of cutting at each stage, apparently changes the original material in some unknown way. But the preparation is so tedious and so different from anything in standard science that chemists do not deign to investigate its mechanism.

To form the next decimal potency, one part of this dilution is then mixed with nine parts more neutral medium and shaken or triturated. The third decimal potency is made with one part of the second decimal and nine more parts neutral medium. At this point the original substance has become only one-thousandth of the final pill.

There is another common scale in which the dilutions are made, with one part substance and *ninety-nine* parts neutral medium; in fact, this, and not the prior more substantial scale, is most commonly used in triturations. The third centesimal dilution produces a pill with one-millionth part of the original medicine. If poison nut were the selected tincture for its tendency to produce symptoms like the symptoms of a disease, then the nut juice would constitute one-millionth of the actual medicine at the third centesimal dilution. By the twelfth centesimal dilution (or twenty-fourth decimal dilution), there is almost certainly no trace of the original substance in most of the medicine, no trace at all (!). No poison nut juice in the remedy called "poison nut," no cuttlefish ink in the remedy called *"Sepia,"* no mercury in the *"Mercury,"* no gold in the *"Aurum,"* no dog's milk in *"Lac Caninum."*

In their 1967 paper "Microdose Paradox: A New Biophysical Concept," G. P. Barnard of Surrey, England, and James H. Stephenson of New York City write:

"In Great Britain, the dilution stages extend to 1000 on the centesimal basis, that is, a 'dilution' of 10^{-2000}. In the U.S.A., the dilution stages are continued to 'dilutions' of $10^{-20,000,000}$. Obviously, any therapeutic practice based on the use of dilutions of these orders of magnitude is manifestly absurd, unless the specific method of preparing these dilutions fortuitously exposes a natural phenomenon of profound biological significance."[45] The only explanation for medicinal activity could be the sequence and method of preparation rather than the raw potency of the molecular substances of the original solute.

To assume that there is any original substance left after homeopathic preparation would be in violation of either Avogadro's Law or some other law of physical chemistry. Avogadro's Law itself is a mainstay of physical science. Proposed originally by the nineteenth-century Italian physicist Count Amadeo Avogadro, it states that the number of molecules in a gram molecular weight of a substance is 6.0225×10^{23}. The 6.0225 is not the key here, but 10^{23} is. For, if a substance is diluted beyond 10^{-24}, with uniform mixing at each stage, there is in all probability nothing left of it in the sample used to prepare the medicine. Each dilution reduces the number of molecules of the substance, which begins at the unimaginably high figure of, roughly, six followed by twenty-three zeros, until by the twenty-fourth decimal dilution (one to nine each time), there should not be a single molecule remaining in any one pill. No doubt, if one or more hung on from irregular mixing, they would be in mortal jeopardy in the passage from the twenty-fourth to the twenty-fifth decimal. Even at dilutions significantly less than 10^{23} substances should have difficulty imposing any chemical activity. In ranges of 10^{-4}, chemists using advanced analytical techniques find traces of virtually every naturally occurring element in the periodic table (though these "contaminants" are admittedly not intentionally introduced or "derived by controlled dilution stages from a saturated solution"[46]). The background impurity level approaches the dilution level of the substance on which the solution is based. Yet the homeopathic preparation has just begun!

This process continues, usually to the thirtieth decimal, but often as far as the one-millionth centesimal, and there is no reason to assume it should stop there. This amount of dilution is beyond comprehension. There is nothing left at the twelfth centesimal, and yet that substance continues to be diluted, one to a hundred, one to a hundred, one to a hundred, almost a million times more to produce the millionth centesimal. Furthermore, there is another scale, called the millesimal, in which substances are serially diluted one part to fifty thousand of neutral medium up into the hundreds of thousands of times. It is worse than putting a sugar cube in the ocean. A bewildered Abraham Lincoln called it the "medicine of a shadow of a pigeon's wing."

As Whitmont puts it,

> Apparently, what we confront here is not a dilution in the ordinary sense, but another, as yet unknown, dispersion of the substance which while "dematerializing" on the molecular level preserves its specific dynamic characteristics and intensifies its energetic charge.[47]

Each dilution, according to homeopaths, *increases* the effective power of the original substance. A reliable homeopathic physician would not think of using the ten-thousandth decimal, let alone the one-millionth centesimal, except in the case of severe deep-seated illness. It is no wonder that homeopathy finds little acceptance in mainstream medicine. Convinced homeopaths have expressed dismay at the bizarre principles of their own pharmacy. Many secretly believe that the working of the medicines is impossible and unbelievable. They go on practicing *only* because they somehow get cures. James Gorman writes:

> In the end, you are left with a puzzle—experiments of disputed value, anecdotal evidence. The anecdotes are most suggestive. Why, after all, do so many patients and doctors have so many accounts of successful treatment with homeopathic medicines? Are they making the stories up? Are all of the accounts examples of the placebo effect? In fact, it is quite curious that the placebo effect is so maligned: regular physicians scoff at homeopathy, saying it's *merely* the placebo effect. Proponents of homeopathy insist that the positive results they see cannot be *merely* the placebo effect.[48]

The mystery of how homeopathic remedies work is reflected in the variety of injunctives given to patients. Most homeopathic doctors believe that certain strong substances can antidote a remedy immediately or at least lessen its curative effects over time. These relapsing agents include allopathic drugs, recreational drugs (marijuana, cocaine, LSD, etc.), megadoses of vitamins, camphor, caffeine, food or drink within fifteen minutes of taking a remedy, electric blankets, and dental drilling. Thus, patients are urged to avoid chocolate, cola, Kahlua, Australian tea tree oil, pau d'arco tea, BenGay, Vick's, Sea Breeze, Chapstick, Noxzema, Tiger Balm, etc. Even doctors who believe all or some of these substances interfere with therapeutic responses to homeopathic medicines set wide ranges for the degree necessary for devitalization. In one patient the remedy can be palliated by one sip of coffee; another must drink several cups a day for nine months before there is a negative effect. Yet one would imagine a great deal of irreversible tissue change from the original potency over nine months. Is this then undermined by coffee? Some homeopaths insist it is. Others deny that any common molecular substance can impede or reverse a nonmolecular, spiritualized effect.

In response to my query about this area of contradicting belief systems, Jonathan Shore told me, "The remedy is like a new seedling. At first, it is easily uprooted or washed away. Later it develops strong root systems and clings tenaciously to the body's tissues."[49]

Another doctor regularly treated animals, with the same success, mainly to reassure himself that his treatment was not just suggestibility plus placebo.

In the physical world, some substances are poisonous, some are nutritious, some are inactive in the human body. Yet after homeopathic "potentization," the majority of these physical properties disappear and new properties occur that are unknown in chemistry. Although there is a rough resemblance between the behavior of a potentized substance and its raw physical base, the differences are great enough to establish a whole new system of what could only be called hermetic medicinal chemistry. Whitmont provides some of its more spectacular characteristics:

> It has been found that the medicinal properties of substances in their high potencies are immediately transferred to the walls of containers as well as to any inert substance upon contact. In many instances, particularly in life-threatening situations, the therapeutic effect of the potentized medicine has been observed to occur with a simultaneity that could not well be accounted for

by physical absorption. I myself once observed a patient in deep coma subsequent to a stroke return to consciousness within minutes after placing a dose of the thousandth potency of *Opium* under her tongue (opium poisoning induces coma).

This phenomenon strikes me as less like digestive absorption than like an exchange of information or a conveying of a "memory" of specific dynamic characteristics in a field process, analogous to the "morphic resonance fields" that Rupert Sheldrake has described.[50]

Elsewhere he writes more metaphorically about the relation between potentization of matter and psychosomatic transformation:

> As substance is disrupted and made chaotic, vibratory rate and transcendental awareness are raised so as to reach into the realm of implicate archetypal order. We might see this as an analogy to the human processes of maturing and aging and the "potentizing" effects of dissipative, disturbing illness and catastrophic factors that "succuss," shake up, our personal lives. They disorder and break up existing inertial structure, upset and confuse our materially encoded sense of order and existence. If and when we can attentively live through this process, a refinement and differentiation of consciousness, tolerance and emotional wisdom and love can be achieved, one that reaches out toward the "telos," to the individuation goal of one's life.[51]

The potentized form of matter, as described by homeopathy, is a unique and stable state, different from gas, liquid, solid, or plasma. Thus, it is theoretically possible to potentize any substance. In actuality, some substances are preferred, for they were in herbal and medicinal use for centuries before homeopathy was formulated. But experimental homeopathy continues to examine the possibility of potentizing new substances and learning their properties as medicines—from their toxicology in material doses to their spiritual vibration in microdoses. This is done not only in the search for materials with unknown therapeutic qualities, but in response to the natural adjustment of pharmacy to a world in which both human and environmental chemistry are changing. The philosophy of esoteric homeopathy demands in fact that the world continue to produce new forms of illness and simultaneously new medicines to treat them.

This would happen whether homeopathic science existed or not.

Furthermore, as homeopathy is practiced in new regions, different local substances become available. For instance, after a disciple of Hahnemann brought homeopathy to India in the middle of the nineteenth century, local provings contributed panther, tiger, and leopard (at least temporarily) to the medicine chest.

A special class of medicines, prepared from bacteria and pathological tissues, was added in the early twentieth century. The nosodes, as these are called, include such initially dismaying substances as bacteria taken from bowels and gonorrheal and syphilitic discharges. More recently, homeopathic experimenters have potentized cat hair, tobacco, opium, cocaine, media exposed to X-ray or sun, HIV virus, their own sperm, sulphur dioxide, and LSD—in each case following the loose homeopathic rule that a substance which brings about an imbalance or pathology in material form is a possible remedy in potentized form.

Clearly, the original physical substance is quickly diluted into nonexistence and passes from the picture. In the case of bacteria and strong poisons, this is fortunate and reassuring. If anything remains after the substance is gone, it must be in the form of a message, a message that has already been passed to the neutral medium before the dilution destroys its source. Perhaps the tincture transfers something like a template of itself or some of its properties to the surrounding solution, much in the way DNA and messenger RNA exchange information in the duplication of living cells. The succussion (shaking) of the tincture after each dilution may "hammer" the message in, and then each successive dilution, with continued succussion, would serve to charge the message, increasing its volume, potency by potency. We initially seem to be left with tiny, white, chemically neutral balls, but if anything like the above occurs, we would also have the vitalized record of a potency. That record would contain not the chemical properties of animal, plant, or mineral, but something that precedes their manifestation and generates it, even as the invisible core disease precedes the visible symptomology.

The so-called microdose phenomenon is not limited to homeopathy. Morphogenetic changes during the embryological development of organisms result from extremely small concentrations of substances. Protein manufacture by RNA transfer itself arises from the positions of single amino acids in long, repetitive chains. Enzymes in minute amounts also catalyze protein and tissue organization. Trace minerals such as selenium have distinct biological effects in the range of a few parts in 10^8. Fluorine to prevent tooth decay is added to public drinking water in amounts of 1 to 10^6. Even medicinal springs do not bear significantly greater mineral content than this.

Gorman made his own survey of nonexplanations in *The New York Times Magazine* article:

> Thierry R. Montfort, president of Boiron [the largest homeopathic manufacturer in the world], says, "We still don't know how to explain the mechanism of action." Beverly Rubik, director of the Center for Frontier Sciences at Temple University, which publishes research on homeopathy, acknowledges, "Nobody knows how it works." There is only speculation on the mechanism of action. Dana Ullman . . . suggests that even in the lowest doses, "something remains: the essence of the substance, its resonance, its energy, its pattern." He also mentions a possible interaction with the life force "similar to what the Chinese call chi." According to Rubik, the homeopathic "signal" may be "informational and electromagnetic in nature."[52]

Ullman describes a recent brouhaha around microdoses:

> In 1988, an article by respected French immunologist Dr. Jacques Benveniste was published in *Nature* that created a whirlwind of controversy.[53] A study which was replicated 70 times in a total of six laboratories at four different universities showed that microdoses of an antigen diluted 1:10 up to 120 times had a significant effect on white blood cells called basophils. Because basophils are known to increase in number when exposed to an antigen, the researchers conjectured that homeopathic doses of an antigen would affect basophils.
>
> In a story that is probably familiar to people who follow controversies in science, *Nature* editor John Maddox, magician James Randi, and NIH researcher Walter Stewart went to the lab which originated the research at the University of Paris South.[54] Although

this lab and others had worked on this research for five years, the *Nature* team felt that they had debunked this original research after their two days of study.

The press never reported on some crucial specifics of this debunking. The research which supposedly debunked Benveniste's work was conducted blind a total of four times. The first time the experiment worked just as the original researchers predicted. This successful experiment was never described or discussed in the press. The next three times, however, the experiment did not show any action of the microdose on the basophils. The press only reported on the three negative outcomes.

When a more stringently controlled trial was recently completed, the press ignored it, with the exception of the *New Scientist* which reported favorably on it.[55] This new experiment was published in the *Journal of the French Academy of Science*.[56] An important, new feature to this experiment was that the researchers first tested the blood samples to make certain that they were sensitive to crude doses of an antigen. Because this experiment was testing allergy hypersensitivity to a specific substance and because not all blood samples will show this sensitivity in regular crude doses, this additional feature to the experiment was essential. As it turned out, 39% of those blood samples which had the sensitivity to crude doses responded to homeopathic doses of an antigen, while 0% of the control group responded.[57]

Science characterized the event-sequence as follows:

In the 30 June issue of *Nature*, French chemist Jacques Benveniste and co-workers published the results of a series of experiments that seemed to have no physical explanation. The researchers measured the response of a type of human white blood cell to varying concentrations of a particular type of antibody. They diluted the antibodies with distilled water to the point where there should have been no antibody molecules left in the solution, and still they observed a reaction from the white blood cells. Standard theory offers no explanation for such a result, and the researchers suggested that the antibodies were somehow leaving an imprint on the water molecules that triggered the response of the white blood cells.

To convince *Nature* to accept the paper, Benveniste arranged for independent laboratories in Israel, Italy, and Canada to repeat the experiments, and researchers from these three labs were listed as co-authors on the final work. The journal held up publication of the paper for two years as it pushed for various substantiations, and finally published it with the condition that later an investigative team would watch Benveniste's group perform the experiments and file a report on the conduct of the work.

That report, which takes up four pages in the 28 July issue, damns Benveniste's experiments as "statistically ill-controlled, from which no substantial effort has been made to exclude systematic error, including observer bias, and whose interpretation has been clouded by the exclusion of measurements in conflict with the claims [of the researchers]." The investigating team depicts the experiment as one whose results were more likely due to the desires of the experimenters than to physical reality. The report suggests that the research team members, two of whom are doctors of homeopathy, wanted the experiments to succeed because that success would support some of the tenets of homeopathic medicine, which uses very small doses of various substances to cure ills.

Maddox said that Randi, who has made a name for himself uncovering trickery of various sorts, was included on the team because Maddox suspected some of the results might be due to fraud. "We thought it quite probable that there was someone in Benveniste's lab who was playing a trick on him," Maddox said. Randi found no evidence of conscious fraud, however, and Maddox said a more likely source of Benveniste's results was "auto-suggestions"—one or more of the researchers seeing what they expected to see or wished to see. Benveniste, replying to the report in the same issue of *Nature*, denounces the behavior and the conclusions of what he calls the "almighty anti-fraud and heterodoxy squad." He notes that neither Randi, Maddox, or Stewart has a background in immunology and claims that this ignorance caused various mistakes and misunderstandings in the investigation. More seriously, he charges that the investigation was more a witch hunt than a sober search for scientific truth. "This was nothing but a real scientific comedy, a parody of an investigation carried out by a magician and a scientific prosecutor working in the purest style of the witches of Salem or of McCarthyist or Soviet ideology," he told the French newspaper *Le Monde*.[58]

A number of reports mention how James Randi turned the investigation into a farce with distracting magic tricks and performance of smug disinterest and exhibitionism.

Benveniste is quoted in *The Los Angeles Times* of July 27, 1988:

> We have always said there was a possibility of an error of methodology and that possibility is still open. I will certainly have these experiments done again.... Never, but never ... let these people get in your lab. Scientists must not be treated like criminals.[59]

This dispute will certainly recur for decades until we have both the tools and disposition to resolve it. At a time of global pollution and resource consumption, we could certainly use a science of energy which continues to produce more from less and leads us into a future of sustainable technologies *ad infinitum*. If microdoses work, then substances in nature contain an unknown, profound, powerful, bottomless, and benign energy having to do with atomic energy or nuclear fission.

Whatever their definition, homeopathic medicines cannot be considered substance-based drugs: they are parallels, vibrations, spiritual entities, intelligences, messages. They are qualities of substance, not quantities.

Ullman has been a clearinghouse for innovative paradigms to get homeopaths out of their vitalistic *cul de sac*.

> Quantum physics may help lay the theoretical foundations for how the homeopathic microdoses act. Bell's Theorem, an integral part of quantum physics, holds that things are fundamentally interconnected and inseparable. Various studies have concluded that interconnections exist and that some things can dramatically affect other things, even if only very small changes in one thing take place and even if these things are great distances from each other. Quantum physicists do not precisely know the nature of these interconnections, but some evidence suggests that homeopathy's Law of Similars and its use of infinitesimal doses is additional confirmation of this mysterious but real phenomenon.
>
> The diluted homeopathic medicines may have distinct effects upon the diluent (water) even in extreme high dilutions. What

this means and the implications of this on homeopathy is that the dilutions, even beyond Avogadro's number, may not erase the template or the memory of the original drug once it has been registered as present as a particle in a solution. The medicine may then have a "field effect" upon the solution in which it is being diluted and ultimately have a field effect upon the entire organism who imbibes it.

Macroscopic changes can occur in living organisms when specific key enzymes, hormones, or tissues are activated, even if only slightly activated. Modern chaos theory tends to support this observation. One of the basic assumptions of chaos theory is that minute changes can lead to huge differences.

It is presently recognized that living and non-living things have their own resonance. As science writer K. C. Cole wrote, "Planets and atoms and almost everything in between vibrate at one or more natural frequencies. When something else nudges them periodically at one of those frequencies, resonance results."[60] Cole goes on to say that resonance means to resound, to sound again, or to echo, and the power of resonance is in the pushing or pulling in the same direction that the force is already going. A synchrony of small pushes can add up to create a significant change. A classic example of the force of resonance is witnessed in the phenomenon of soldiers walking in place over a bridge, causing it to collapse. . . .

An article in *Gastroenterology*[61] has suggested that small doses may have a more significant effect than large doses because of a "therapeutic window." Such action is more likely when an organism is in a state of "metastable excitation," a hypersensitive state which is "cocked and ready to go" as soon as a specific stimulus triggers the avalanche effect. The homeopathic Law of Similars may be ultimately the link to finding a substance in nature, which when individually prescribed, can trigger this avalanche effect.

Using small doses of the wrong substance or the right substance at the wrong time creates little or no effect. This is why the incorrect homeopathic medicine doesn't do anything.

What is also interesting about resonance is that resonance is more powerful when there is a little friction—when the force is similar to though not exactly the same as the initial force. The resonance becomes broader, creating something similar to a chord rather than a single note. The relationship of these ideas to healing is that homeopaths find that the most effective homeopathic medicine is one that is the "most similar," not necessarily the "same" as the symptoms the person is experiencing.[62]

This would explain why homeopathy is not allergology or isopathy. It involves a complex set of multidimensional harmonics rather than a linear relationship of antibodies and antigens.

In 1900 Kent wrote:

> Vital disorder cannot be turned into order except by something similar in quality to the vital force. It is not similitude in quantity that we want, in weights and measures, but it is similarity in quality, in power, in plane, that must be sought for.
>
> Medicines, therefore, cannot affect the high and interior planes of the physical economy unless they are raised to the plane of similarity in quality. The individual who needs *Sulphur* in the very highest degrees may take *Sulphur* sufficient to move his bowels, may rub it upon the skin, may wear it in his stockings, can take *Sulphur* baths, all without effect upon his disease. In that form the drug is not in correspondence with his sickness, it does not affect him in the same plane in which he is sick, and so it cannot affect the cause and flow from thence to the circumference.[63]

When I asked Theodore Enslin about this phenomenon[64] he singled out the high potencies, the nonmaterial dilutions, which, he said, "are a division of energy in the sense that the low ones are not. Up to six or seven X, there is a recognizable amount of molecular structure left in the pill. In the high potencies, it's not substance at all; it depends entirely on a release of energy. Energy is divisible, but it's not divisible in the same sense that molecular substance is. These potencies are really quite dangerous. A good physician prescribing can give a high potency and in one dose clear up something that has resisted all kinds of prescribing for years, and it seems miraculous. Anyone handling that had better be pretty competent. I mean, there are things that no good physician would deny, that are not known so far as those things are concerned. Substances that have absolutely no effect in low potencies suddenly have a very high one in the high potencies. And they usually are far more marked mentally than any other way. The one that is the old warhorse of the thing is *Silicea*, which is nothing more than flint.

In a low potency you can take flint, you can eat rocks until they make a hole in your stomach, and it will have no medicinal effect whatsoever. But suddenly you get *Silicea* at 30x or higher; you can take it to the CM [the one-hundred-thousandth centesimal], which is the ultimate, and it has a profound mental effect, something that is not present in the lower potencies."

A 1974 publication of the American Institute of Homeopathy puts this in quasi-pharmaceutical language:

> The homoeo-discipline is concerned with the specific, the individual, the distinctive. In order to achieve that goal, the homoeo-medical discipline endeavours to study the reaction of the organism to an incitant and not the action of the drug itself. In doing so it reverses the roles of organism and drug and places emphasis on the vital response. . . .
>
> The point we wish to make is that the homoeo-discipline denies that the drug possesses any power or virtue, but postulates that contact between the drug and the living organism sets in motion an influence. The drug is not injected, digested, assimilated, or transported physically. In and of itself it can do nothing except under the highly specific circumstances: when the properties of sensitivity, irritability, idiosyncrasy are exquisitely developed, the vital reaction—which is a function of the host and not of the agent—takes place.[65]

Not of the agent! That sums up the homeopathic paradox. What does the Food and Drug Administration think? Gorman checked this out:

> Homeopathic medicines are considered drugs by the FDA but minimally regulated. By law, all new drugs must be tested for safety and efficacy. So far the FDA has chosen not to enforce this provision for homeopathic drugs, because their harmlessness is generally accepted. In 1988 the FDA did issue labeling and packaging guidelines, and defined what homeopathic drugs could be sold over the counter (essentially, those marketed for what are called self-limiting conditions, like the common cold). Although many critics challenge the efficacy of homeopathic remedies, to date the FDA has chosen not to give them priority. Daniel L. Michels, director of the Office of Compliance of the FDA's Center for Drug Evaluation and Research, emphasizes that this hands-off approach "is not to say these products are effective."

Perhaps the most vocal critic of homeopathy is William T. Jarvis, president of the National Council Against Health Fraud, an organization that is death on everything from health food to acupuncture. Jarvis says proponents of homeopathy are either "stupid" or "deliberately fraudulent." Claiming that "the FDA has let the public down" by failing to make homeopathic medicines prove their safety and efficacy as do other drugs, he says, "If we had the money we would sue them." *Consumer Reports* has also called for testing of homeopathic medicines.[66]

The ostensible success of homeopathic medicine has always suggested avenues of research to unconventionally minded biologists and physicists. Thus, new models for the activity of succussed microdoses have continued to be explored. In 1996 scientists at American Technologies Group in California found that a previously unknown type of stable crystal was formed when substances diluted in distilled water were shaken or stirred and then rediluted and reshaken. Shaped like lentil beans in flat-disc configurations and aggregating in clusters from 15 nm. to several microns across, these entities were named I_E crystals by physicist Shui-Yin Lo (for "ice/electrical-field"), though they are different from ice in geometrical shape, charge, and density.[67] "What's additionally interesting and initially confusing," adds Dr. Lo, "is that the number of ice crystals actually increases as does their biological and chemical effect after each time we dilute and shake the water."[68] In fact, diluting and shaking increased the amount of crystals in solution from approximately 1–2 percent to 10 percent.

The I_E crystals appear to carry information and remain stable even at temperatures above one hundred degrees, continually breaking apart and reforming by dipole interaction, producing more numerous and larger crystals. To achieve this shearing, fragmenting, and crystallizing effect takes vigorous shaking—something like homeopathic succussion; simple chemical agitation will not accomplish it.

I_E crystals have thus far been used as additives to decrease smog and carbon build-up in engines and improve fuel efficiency. They have also reduced scaling and fouling in ethylene crackers (large plastic-manufacturing furnaces) and other heat-transfer equipment. Some scientists have found that they have a positive biological effect on fungal and bacterial strains—an increase in titers of microorganism-generated enzymes and a decrease in fermentation time.

Lo acknowledges the unresolved relationship of these crystals to homeopathic microdoses:

> The homeopaths were definitely onto something, but our discovery of I_E crystals may help their medicines become even more powerful, and these I_E crystals will probably have significant industrial applications, energy-transfer benefits, cleansing uses, and ecological protection. . . . There seems to be something unique there in water that undergoes extreme dilution, and we now have the laboratory evidence and even the photographic evidence to verify it. Thus far, we have only systematically tested substances that have been diluted one-to-ten thirteen times. Homeopathic doctors sometimes use medicines which are diluted one-to-ten thirty, two hundred, a thousand, or more times, and we have not tested these extreme dilutions yet. However, I would not be surprised if I_E crystals are also observed in these doses. Based on our research to date, every dilution beyond the sixth has found I_E crystals in them.[69]

6. Psychomorphology

Some homeopaths have attempted to establish links between substances and their microdose effects. The pioneer in such attempts, Edward Whitmont, is perhaps uniquely qualified by his combined practice of homeopathy and archetypal psychology. Beginning in the 1940s, he wrote a series of speculative articles on the various remedies, arguing, in essence, that the underlying vitality that gives rise to the shape or character of the entity from which each remedy is extracted also gives rise to its cohesive healing virtue.

Whitmont proposes that pharmacy and psychology are linked on a profound psychosomatic level. When we concretize medicinal virtues in remedies or intuit curative relationships, we are discovering associations that already objectively exist in the world of nature. The dynamic totality of nature brings together events and images according to their own essential natures. According to Whitmont, "Even as the symbol is the image and expression, in terms of form and appearance, of specific psychic energies, so is the morphological manifestation or appearance of an objective function in nature the expression and image in the world of sense perception of its intrinsic functional dynamism."[70]

The Doctrine of Signatures describes relationships which the Doctrine of Similars miniaturizes and transposes to a submolecular realm. Dog's Milk, Poison Oak, White Cedar, and Silver are medicines for reasons we may intuitively grasp through the mute synchronicity we share with them and through qualities expressed in both them and us at different levels of structure in nature. Our link is fractal and cybernetic. Neither their morphology nor our morphology is accidental; thus our connections are, in some sense, authentic as signified. The discovery of homeopathic virtues, like the discovery of the DNA helix and the meiosis of cells, is not accidental, for we are intrinsic and organized by the same order and under the same terms. Ancient herbal and animal medicines come likewise from a psyche which is cosmic and collective and includes the structure of botanical and animal forms in its "meaning" even if these lie outside the more limited mind-psyche of science.

Carl Jung writes:

> The assumption that the human psyche possesses layers that lie *below* consciousness is not likely to arouse serious opposition. But that there could just as well be layers lying *above* consciousness seems to be a surmise which borders on a *crimen laesae majestatis humanae.* In my experience the conscious mind can only claim a relatively central position and must put up with the fact that the unconscious psyche transcends and as it were surrounds it on all sides. Unconscious contents connect it backwards with physiological states on the one hand and archetypal data on the other. But it is extended *forward* by intuitions which are conditioned partly by archetypes and partly by subliminal perceptions depending on the relativity of time and space in the unconscious.[71]

To Jung, the objective psyche could transcend space and time and embody the clandestine meaning of any substance, not just its medicinal virtue. But Jung never translated integers or biological morphologies into absolutes; only the unknowable archetypes are true absolutes—any manifestation of them is fluid. At Jung's personal suggestion, Whitmont tried to arrive at a more reliable system of relationships combining psychology and substance.

For Whitmont, the potentized medicines embody archetypes that also shape the plants, animals, and minerals—in fact, all of nature. If one can tap the essence of anything, not its procreative seed or crystal *per se* but its elemental source, then medicinal action can be liberated on the same plane. Stones, diseases, metals, bacteria, even human symbols are equivalent on this level. The impulse which gives rise to the precise form of an oak tree or an eel, under highly individual environmental-embryological blueprints, gives rise under different circumstances to an ulcer, a virus, pottery, a myth, a phobia, a potency, etc.

Whitmont explains the underlying psychosomatic unity:

> It is as though all of our problems, disturbances and complexes also portrayed themselves in some form of explicate earth-substance-imperfection. Implicate order encodes or explicates itself in our psyches as complexes: as image, emotion and drive patterns that, through their "incarnations," manifest as conditioned deviations from the archetypal "ideal." (Father, mother, love, hate, transition, heroic fight, surrender, permeability, etc.) They incarnate likewise in the patterns of biological life energies and in the forms of animal, plant and mineral substances.
>
> These correspondences are not of a linear one-to-one nature, however. A father crisis, for instance, does not correspond to a particular substance. The patterns are more comprehensive and their connections far from clear to us. A parental problem that activates a crisis in the realm of permeability—when it is a matter of defining one's boundaries, physically or psychologically—may, for instance, correspond to allergic states and to a calcium process. When the resistance of one's "fiber" is in need of restructuring it may correspond to silicon or pulsatilla, the windflower. It may be "similar" to *Hepar sulfuris* (calcium sulfide) when the issue is one of an interplay between imbalanced permeability (calcium) and "fiery" uncontrollable overreaction (sulfur) that expresses itself in inflammatory conditions. A tremendous amount of study and research is still necessary to clarify these areas. We have as yet too little understanding of the qualitative aspects of the substances that structure our world. Until now we have studied only *quan-*

titative compositions—the chemistry of minerals, plants and animal life, but, short of the homeopathic provings, have never yet systematically concerned ourselves with the qualitative "moods," "personalities" or "souls" (anthropomorphic terms for lack of more adequate ones that would refer to *their* life forces, Qi and "astral"-emotional fields) of the elements of our surroundings, let us say of antimony, silver, the bushmaster snake, quartz or a gentian or poison ivy plant, or with the "soul" of our cosmos.[72]

The intuition here is that each substance will naturally reflect some aspect of its potential healing archetype in its habitat, chemistry, affinities, and growth patterns. Homeopathic remedies are then sublimated from the tinctures of these plants, animals, minerals, and other material and reduced to the archetypal plane, i.e., dematerialized so that they are in tune with the disease as archetype rather than as pathology.

Whitmont calls these quanta "psychosomatic wholes," "dynamic totalities"; they exist simultaneously in nature and psyche, complementarily in medicine and myth. Some characteristic of a plant, animal, or mineral must persist in the character of its disease and its remedy. In discussing *Sepia,* for instance, Whitmont draws our attention to "the dynamic meaning of the shell-enclosed jelly."[73] This has a symbolic relationship to the alchemical vessel of prima materia, which is also the uterus, and the feminine receptacle of the self in both sexes. *Sepia* may then project a healing function for equivalent disorders in either personality or physiological process.

Whitmont continues:

> Even as a half of the cuttlefish's body must remain within the enclosing shell, in spite of all attempts to break loose, so also the temperamental, sexual and emotional tendencies which one would disown cannot simply be cast off; they can only be slowly and gradually transformed by developing a conscious understanding with which to complement the world of instinctive feeling which is woman's primary expression and experience. Wherever the gradual expansion gives way to a violent, protesting attitude, suppression takes the place of gradual transformation and pathology arises. Challenge to and suppression of the quiet, contemplative and receptive feminine qualities, symbolized by the "creative vessel," thus become the keynotes of the *Sepia* pathology.[74]

This is not necessarily itself the *Sepia* illness, but it is, conceivably, the underlying psychosomatic message which precedes the onset of pathology. Whitmont mentions the irritable, fault-finding, spiteful quality of *Sepia*; the movement from antagonism to gentleness and affection, the oversensitivity, the premature aging. These come from a suppressed unconscious personality, which has a concrete somatization simultaneously in a mollusk and *Sepia*.

The *Natrum Muriaticum* patient, the one whose disease is "salt," is inconsolable for a reason having to do with failure of basic assimilation of vital energies, hence disintegration of life forming in the seed.[75]

The *Phosphorus* patient is ecstatic but terrified of a coming darkness, speedy but easily exhausted, somehow stunted in growth and anemic.[76] But then *Phosphorus* also contains within it an extreme brightness, a luminescence that is not radioactive but oxidating.

Rudolf Hauschka writes:

> *Phosphorus* . . . shines and pours out light, but is also a condensing agent. . . . Nerves are built of protein high in phosphorus. Indeed, the nervous system as a whole is as clear a revelation of the phosphorus process as the circulatory system is of the aluminum process. *Phosphorus* flames give light, but are cold. Our nervous system endows us with the cool, clear light of consciousness; but it is also the transmitting agent for the formative impulses that shape the body's plastic organs.
>
> The phosphorus process co-operates on the one hand with the silica in our skin, on the other with lime in our bony structure. The skin contains innumerable nerve-endings, which convey impressions of the world around us. Though silica creates skin surfaces, it is the phosphorus process that gives them surface sensitivity. It is to phosphorus that we owe awareness of our bodies and a bodily consciousness of selfhood. The skin, with its nerve inclusions, thus forms a boundary between world and individual.[77]

The diseases treated with homeopathic *Phosphorus* include ones of the nervous system, especially left-sided symptoms, which suggest the unconscious hemisphere of the brain; gastrointestinal irritations, including lightheadedness and desire for cold water which is then vomited; liver cirrhosis; diabetes; and general tubercular conditions.

The person suffering from *Phosphorus* is nauseated by the fragrance of flowers when too strong; he is extremely jumpy, sensitive to touch, and disturbed by thunderstorms' phosphoric energy.

With *Lycopodium*, Whitmont focuses on its habits as a creeping moss whose spores "do not moisten as they repel water . . . are extremely hard but burn with a very bright flash when ignited . . . germinate only after 6–7 years."[78] The *Lycopodium* patient has high nervous tension, is developed mentally but with a weak body. He craves open air and loosens tight clothing; he is dry, constipative, and noneliminative, with kidney and urinary symptoms. His diseases progress slowly and inwardly, with a tendency toward cancerous growth. He is bloated and does not digest well; he has bad circulation and lacks inner heat. Is this the symptomology locked in the club moss spore until its archetype is realized in a disease and its potentized substance is used as a remedy? If so, club moss has a prehuman personality, expressed in both a disease and a medicine.

Whitmont emphasizes, alternately, the physical manifestation of each substance, its makeup as a plant or animal or mineral, and its meaning in human symbolism and myth. For instance, with *Lachesis,* rattlesnake poison, he notes the serpent as the dark, underground function, the figure which, in Gnostic tradition, replaces Christ on the cross: "The serpent pathology is the unintegrated life impulse, the unintegrated libido, the unintegrated instinct split off and split in itself . . . *Lachesis* is the penalty of unlived life."[79] Thus the *Lachesis* patient is egotistic, vicious, sexually repressive, and mean, all in frustration for the actual self not lived. The person has intense pain everywhere, cramps, pressure, sensitivity, swollen gums and toothaches, extreme excitability with irritation and disease in the sexual organs, especially the ovaries.

Sulphur is decayed and putrefied earth, but in alchemical terms, it is a ferment which is the source of fire and gold and can be transformed by the mutative process into spirit and soul.[80] The *Sulphur* personality is characterized by skin eruptions, general congestion and stagnation; it contains raw uncomplicated psora, with a tendency to dirtiness, distraction, unfocused genius, and mental brilliance with disregard for personal being.

One physician concluded a diagnosis with the following assessment:

> Gold is an interesting thing in the history of man. It has been hoarded as wealth. People have worn it as jewelry and struggled for possession of it. It is associated with the sun. It is found often in quartz, and near the surface of the ground. Pans in rivers trap gold particles. It is purple in the colloidal state and used for staining glass in cathedrals. Gold anchors the value of money systems. Without the anchor, value disintegrates. *You* have a disease called *Aurum*, gold. I will give you its medicine.[81]

In terms of the rational mind or of any usual system of mind / body, the remedy is ridiculous. In archetypal terms linking man, woman, mineral, and nature, it is a powerful characterization.

Homeopathy almost becomes psychoanalysis in the way that it dramatizes its cures in vivid, evocative character types. An astute homeopath conceivably transmits some aspect of her remedies in a linguistic, imagistic portrayal of them, timed to startle the patient into self-recognition. The patient comes to embody a remedy as he or she gradually enacts it by considering and then performing answers to a doctor's idiosyncratic and personal.questions. This variant of transference can sometimes be more powerful and efficient than long, protracted psychoanalyses that get caught up in neurotic symptom playbacks and professional advice and miss the singular biophysical essence of a condition.

Homeopathy is also ceremonial in a psychosymbolic way. Doctor and patient participate in a drama of amulets (crystallized essences), grails, and narrative mythologies resembling a Navaho sand-painting rite or Aranda cave initiation. A mysterious, archetypal diagnosis is followed by treatment with a spiritualized substance. Some of this may be telepathic or telekinetic in a way that science does not yet recognize; some of it may represent instantaneous field states that move from the universal to the individual through a fortuitous combination of doctor, Repertory, original substance, potentization, vitality of patient, and larger fields like the ones associated with molecular chaos (organizing the giant cyclonic spots on Mars, Saturn, and Neptune) or morphic resonance, which transcends time and space to bring evolving forms into correspondence with one another.

Homeopathy is applied medically in the absence of an answer to these riddles; yet it must be assumed that it has somehow captured enough of the elements of an unknown biophysics to be effective. Most homeopaths would rather repeat a successful formula than try to figure out which of its elements are archaic and decorative, hence possibly superfluous. We end up with a system that is far more lucid in practice than in presentation.

But we must put all this in deeper perspective. What is left for us here, as in all mysteries, is to return to the birthplace in order to understand better what was set loose.

Chapter 4

The Life and Work
of Samuel Hahnemann

Samuel Hahnemann was born at midnight, April 10–11, 1755, in the German town of Meissen, near the Polish and Czechoslovakian borders. The Hahnemann family had migrated from the west a generation earlier so that Samuel's father could work at the local porcelain factory. So-called Dresden china had been originated by Johann Bottger, an alchemist, in 1710, as a distraction from his search for gold, and the Saxon porcelain industry was located at Meissen, on the Elbe River, close to its rich clay beds. A factory was established at Albrecht Castle and in 1743 an art school was added. Writing in his journal at the age of thirty-six, Hahnemann describes his beginnings:

> I was born on April 10th, 1755, in the Electorate of Saxony, one of the most beautiful parts of Germany....
>
> My father, Christian Gottfried Hahnemann, together with my mother Johanna Christiana, *née* Spiess, taught me how to read and write whilst playing. My father ... was a painter for the porcelain factory of [Meissen], and the author of a brief treatise on watercolour painting.[1]

Hahnemann was born also into the centuries of German strife. The Seven Years' War, during which the Prussian King, Frederick II, raided the Saxon porcelain industry, ended in his eighth year, leaving his family impoverished. His homeopathic work shared a horoscope with Napoleon's march across Europe.

More obscurely, Hahnemann was born into a German occult tradition, not by personal study or inclination so much as by his time and place and the nature of his eventual quest. To the south, in Switzerland and Austria, Paracelsus, two hundred and fifty years earlier, and Carl Jung and Rudolf Steiner, one hundred and fifty years later, challenged the mysteries of spirit in matter. Each time, out of a prior riddle, a new riddle formed. Hahnemann did his work in the name of matter, and like the later Austrian physician Wilhelm Reich, came to spirit, to vital energy, only inevitably and by default.

Hahnemann emerged from his adolescence remarkably learned. When his boyhood studies were interrupted by war and his father's demands that he learn a trade, he continued to study on his own, and at age sixteen, was taken into the Prince's School in Meissen by the rector, tutoring pupils in Greek and Latin in exchange for tuition. He graduated at twenty with a dissertation (in Latin) on the construction of the human hand, after which he attended Leipzig University.

When he first realized the pitiable state of the medicine of his time, Hahnemann refused to practice it, out of fear of doing more harm than good, and he supported himself only by translating. From the age of thirty to thirty-four, he published over two thousand pages, most of it from non-German sources, with a few conventional articles of his own on sores, ulcers, and drugs. Almost a third of that work was a rendering of the French classic "The Story of Abelard and Heloise" from English into German.

"By teaching German and French to a wealthy young Greek from Jassy in Modavia, as well as by translations from English, I procured for myself for a time the means of subsistence...."[2]

The translations were no small matter. They included physiology texts, descriptions of experiments with copper, a work on hydrophobia, two volumes on mineral waters and warm baths, and various writings on practical medicine. Hahnemann's own earliest creative work emerges from this scholarship. For instance, at twenty-seven, as an amateur chemist, he translated a complex French treatise on industrial chemistry, correcting chemical errors and adding additional techniques in footnotes.

The intellectual impact on Hahnemann of his own prehomeo-pathic work is generally underestimated. There is a reason why homeopathy spoke in refined concepts from the beginning. Its fluency came out of the labyrinth of ancient languages and remote peoples, the ignored work of obscure botanists and physicians of different nations. Hahnemann made a synthesis utterly different from any of its parts.

Much of Hahnemann's research was not entirely medicine or relevant to medicine. But homeopathy was not "medicine" either in any usual sense. It was a theory of nature, humankind, and civilization, as universal and dramatic as Darwinian biology. Translation involves a highly scientific, disciplined meditation on the structure of language, the roots of meaning, and transformations between codes and dialects. Hidden meanings that were invisible in one seamless dialect leap from etymologies. Homeopathy resembles these seminal codes and deep syntactic structures more than it does the concretizations of standard medicine. Hahnemann's rigor is primitive and classical, not progressive.

The founder did not plan to spring "homoeopathy" on the world, but he had the old masters in his head and he knew from experience that contemporary medicine was a disgrace. It was time to return to the drawing board. Greek alchemy, European herbalism, Arabic chemistry, native pharmacies—even though we cannot show their exact contributions to homeopathy—are there, transformed through Hahnemann's synthesis.

It is not as though Hahnemann reapplied old texts to "modern" medicine. He had a new grid by virtue of his time in Europe, plus he did much more than bring back olden wisdom; he reinvented it in a scientific context. In that brief and almost silent hiatus between the end of academic hermeticism and the birth of professional science, he coaxed a single child from their furtive union.

From age thirty-five to thirty-eight, Hahnemann translated medical, agricultural, and chemical books, notably materia medicas from English, French, and Italian. His last such, fourteen years later, in 1806, was the Swiss physician Albrecht von Haller's *Materia Medica of German Plants, Together with Their Economic and Technical Use*, from a French version of the original Latin. Hahnemann's expertise, by this time, included plant names, medical uses of plants, chemical compounds, and various European-language syntax systems. When, in 1810, in his fifty-sixth year, he was required to give a public lecture in order to teach at the Medical Institute in Leipzig, everyone expected a passionate defense of homeopathy. He surprised his audience with a lecture on the ancient medical uses of hellebore, quoting from German, French, English, Italian, Latin, Greek, Hebrew, and Arabic sources, including doctors, herbalists, and natural philosophers. It was a *tour de force* not only in medical theory, but also in botany, etymology, and comparative mythology.

It was, however, in Hahnemann's 1790 translation of the Scottish physician William Cullen's *Treatise on Materia medica* that a new science emerged.

Cullen had a typical, mechanical view of the body. He believed that disease was caused by the variation in the "flux" of nervous energy. As primary organs, like the heart and brain, became blocked and irritated, they communicated this information to other parts of the body, leading to general debility. Nervous ailments were deemed equally mechanical. If they evolved from the direct pressure of agitated blood, for instance, they could be relieved by bloodletting. Pure physical inflammation was treated by either acid or alkaline medicines, the former to counteract an alkaline abundance and the latter to dilute an acid abundance.

Since the body was a mere irritable jelly, the role of medicines in general was to stir up that jelly, stimulate its irritability, and set it into corrective spasm. Cullen's prescriptions were always contraries, in order to redirect the inherent motions of a relatively simple solid. His diagnostic tendency was to reduce the number of diseases to classes of inflammations and blockages and to explain any varying forms as subcategories of the major ones. That way, the number of possible medicines was fixed by the range of spasms necessary to clear the system. The resemblance to homeopathy on the general issue of irritability is not entirely accidental, for Cullen was a follower of Georg Ernst Stahl and the early Montpellier school of Vitalists. It was necessary only for him to replace Stahl's *Anima*, a natural, harmonious, self-corrective healer and regulator, with a more fleshy kind of irritability, to arrive at "Solidism."

Cullen and Hahnemann collide in notes appended to the latter's translation of the former.

Cullen rejects the notion that Peruvian bark (quinine) can have a specific (i.e., unexplained, intrinsic) effect in the treatment of intermittent fever; he says it is just a composite tonic, bringing together the bitter and astringent qualities which combine to give it a power. The translator balks here, and in his footnote to page 108 of Volume II of Cullen's work, he offers a different solution:

> By combining the strongest bitters and the strongest astringents we can obtain a compound which, in small doses, possesses more of both these properties than the bark and yet in all Eternity no fever specific can be made from such a compound. The author should have accounted for this. This undiscovered principle of the effect of the bark is probably not easy to find. Let us consider the following: Substances which produce some kind of fever (very strong coffee, pepper, arnica, ignatia bena, arsenic) counteract these types of intermittent fever. I took, for several days, as an experiment, four drams of good china [cinchona, a quinine source] twice daily. My feet and fingertips, etc., at first became cold; I became languid and drowsy; then my heart began to palpitate; my pulse became hard and quick; an intolerable anxiety and trembling (but without a rigor); prostration in all the limbs; then pulsation in the head, redness of the cheeks, thirst; briefly, all the symptoms usually associated with intermittent fever appeared in succession, yet without the actual rigor.... This paroxysm lasted from two to three hours every time, and recurred when I repeated the dose and not otherwise. I discontinued the medicine and I was once again in good health.[3]

In other words, the remedy had a specific, idiosyncratic, systemic effect, unaccounted for by any of its component properties—Paracelsus' quintessence.

The debut of homeopathy in a footnote reminds us that Hahnemann intended scholarship more than innovation. Healing by medicinal similars was obviously a time-honored way of treating disease. Certainly he had come across it hundreds of times in his reading. To that, he was adding a forceful, anti-rationalist experiment. After all, similars were specifics. The implication was obvious: forget prior categories and test things empirically. He meant to be instructive, but he sounded self-enamored and peevish. Other doctors complained immediately: of what use is such idiosyncratic data? Are we to try all medicines on ourselves at mortal risk?

Hahnemann served in a number of medical positions in his early life, but he always gave them up and returned to translating and research. In 1781, when he was twenty-six, he married the seventeen-year-old daughter of the local apothecary in Gommern, and after working as Medical Officer of Health in Dresden, he moved to Leipzig to be near the university. It was here that Hahnemann translated Cullen, but the real controversy he stirred up was not homeopathic at all.

In 1792 Emperor Leopold II of Austria died while under emergency treatment. Because of the political delicacy of the situation, the three doctors involved issued for publication a full description of the Emperor's illness, its treatment, and the ensuing demise of the patient. Hahnemann responded in a Gotha paper:

> The bulletins state: "On the morning of February 28th, [the Emperor's] doctor, Lagusius, found a severe fever and distended abdomen"—he tried to fight the condition by venesection [bloodletting], and as this failed to give relief, he repeated the process three times more without any better result. We ask, from a scientific point of view, according to what principles has anyone the right to order a second venesection when the first has failed to bring relief? As for a third, Heaven help us!; but to draw blood a fourth time when the three previous attempts failed to alleviate! To abstract the fluid of life four times in twenty-four hours from a man who has lost flesh from mental overwork combined with a long continued diarrhoea, without procuring any relief for him! Science pales before this![4]

This hardly endeared him to the profession.

Hahnemann was, by inclination, a pragmatist and a holist. His Christian and medical asceticism made him scrupulous about life-style and diet. In a time of poor ventilation in houses and lack of concern about contamination, he insisted upon exercise, nutritious meals, running water, and open windows. His vitalism did not dissuade him from intuiting the danger of microbes, toxins, and agents of infection.

The rules of hygiene Hahnemann laid down, though obvious to us, were almost totally unrecognized in his milieu. For instance, he insisted on scraping clean a wound and on bandaging with alcohol-soaked cloths; he actually prescribed fresh air, exercises, cheerful company, warm and cold baths; he recommended that doctors prepare their own medicines and be personally responsible for the continuity of a treatment. Throughout his career, he remained a mixture of the erudite and simple, the dreaming magus and the efficient nurse. He stumbled from the West's ancient books into a hodgepodge of doctors all "born yesterday" and knowing nothing of their traditions. That such pretenders should prepare their own medicines seemed to him ethical and practical, for he had already trained himself in sophisticated laboratory techniques and he had investigated much of the extant history of botany and medicine. He naively assumed others would be willing, if not to do the same, at least to acknowledge its tradition.

It is a telling irony of medical history that the man who seems to stand most against modern germ theory as the primary hypothesis of disease was an early advocate of boiling the utensils used by patients with contagious diseases and isolation of those patients from others (either in a hospital or a private house). He criticized hydrotherapy (cold-water treatment) and mineral baths as ineffective, and standard pharmacy and bloodletting (obviously) as excessive and unhealthy. He ridiculed the standard modes of treatment of mental patients, which combined crude cranial surgery with incarceration. Doctors took the provocative language of mental patients literally and responded to insults with insults, to asocial deeds with punishment. Hahnemann argued that aberrant behavior was a disease, no different from physical ones. Mind/body unity was to be a touchstone of homeopathy.

Hahnemann advocated public health as a desirable civic and personal responsibility and wrote books and pamphlets, in one of which the following exegesis appears:

> In order to have fuel and low rents, several miserable families will often herd together, frequently in one room, and they are careful not to let in any fresh air through window or door, because that might also let in the cold. The animal exhalations

from perspirations and the breath become concentrated, stagnant and foul in these places; one person's lungs do their best to take away from the others all the small amount of life-giving air remaining, exhaling in exchange impurities from the blood. The melancholy twilight of their small, darkened windows is combined with the enervating dampness and musty smell of old rags and rotting straw; fear, envy, quarrelsomeness and other passions do their best to destroy completely what little health there is; all this can only be known by one whose calling has compelled him to enter these hovels of misery. Here contagious epidemics not only go on spreading easily and almost unceasingly if the slightest germ has chanced to fall there, but it is here that they actually originate, break out and become fatal even to more fortunate citizens.[5]

During the years preceding the writing of his *Organon*, Hahnemann remained unsettled and unable to come to terms with professional medicine. After an unsuccessful stint at a mental hospital in Gotha, he spent ten years moving between city and country, attempting to earn a living. His career was marked with brilliant cures but incessant controversy. His insistence on manufacturing his own medicines and practicing in an unorthodox manner alienated both apothecaries and physicians. In one much-publicized case, a certain Prince Schwarzenberg died after leaving Hahnemann's care for the bloodletting of his own physicians. Hahnemann walked in his funeral procession not so much to show respect as to dramatize his conviction of his own innocence in the death.

These were painful times in which he witnessed the illness and death of several of his own children. Having scoured the existing systems of medicine for the needed remedies, he finally concluded, in despair:

"After 1,000 to 2,000 years, then, we are no further!"[6]

What was missing was a logic that explained the variety of diseases and offered a consistent strategy of treatment. The Hippocratics had discovered important medicines, but their science was a mass of contradictions. And medicine since that time had only chased its own questions in self-contradicting, nonproductive circles. No one knew why one disease expressed itself in fever, another in chills, and what the heat of a bath or the spirit of a tonic actually did to a pathology. Hahnemann could not accept Paracelsus' occultism; yet he realized that Paracelsus had practiced the Law of Similars with success, and he took seriously, as a pharmacist, the possibilities of Quintessential remedies while rejecting the alchemical formulas for gold and astrological botany.

More than any of his contemporaries, Hahnemann realized what a profound and complex matter disease was and how unequipped science was to deal with it. The depths of pathology were like the catacombs of history itself, the protean realms of a marvelous and terrifying nature. It *was* the invasion of an unconquerable army, spreading war and poverty and threatening to put all mankind under its dominion. Compared to this enemy, Napoleon was a schoolboy. After all, the invading army was not alien, against man, either; it was the substantial corruption of man's own nature. The devout Christian in Hahnemann led him to associate that corruption with original sin. We no longer use this kind of language, but in the twentieth century we talk, for the first time in scientific terms, about how man is his own enemy and how the illness and iatrogenic "physician" collaborate through millennia to flood society with its inveterate illnesses. Well before Freud, Hahnemann warned that man no longer wanted to be well nor knew how to be, and that planetary survival was itself at stake. He demanded of fellow doctors that they come to their senses before it was too late.

While he was writing the *Organon,* Hahnemann reflected on his path in a letter to a close friend who was a professor of pathology:

> For eighteen years I have been deviating from the ordinary practice of the medical art. . . .
> My sense of duty would not easily allow me to treat the unknown pathological state of my suffering brethren with these unknown medicines. If they are not exactly suitable (and how could the physician know that, since their specific effects had not yet been demonstrated?), they might with their strong potency easily change life into death or induce new disorders and chronic maladies, often more difficult to eradicate than the original disease. The thought of becoming in this way a murderer or a malefactor towards the life of my fellow human beings was most terrible to me, so terrible and disturbing that I wholly gave up

my practice in the first years of my married life. I scarcely treated anybody for fear of injuring him, and occupied myself solely with chemistry and writing.

But then children were born to me, several children, and after a time serious illnesses occurred, which, in tormenting and endangering my children, my own flesh and blood, made it even more painful to my sense of duty that I could not with any degree of assurance procure help for them....Whence then was certain help to be obtained?—was the yearning cry of the comfortless father in the midst of the groaning of his children, dear to him above all else. Night and desolation around me—no sight of enlightenment for my troubled paternal heart.[7]

One might be tempted to presume that Hahnemann wrote in the dark ages before the miracles of technology and microbiology, that we are fortunate to dwell in a subsequent era from which the scourge of disease has been eliminated. However, this would be a fundamental misunderstanding. Yes, Hahnemann observed the diseases caused by the poor hygiene and suppressive medicine of his time. Mercury-dosing, venesection, and escaping sewage led to skin outbreaks, intestinal disorders, neurosis, and epilepsy. Today, our anti-inflammatory drugs, psychotropics, tranquilizers, antibiotics, chemotherapy, immunizations, radiation, and pollution—homeopathically considered—lead to cancer, immune disorders, and new forms of sociopathy. From a Hahnemannian standpoint the underlying problem of medicinal principles has not yet been solved.

In 1796 there appeared, under Hahnemann's authorship, the "Essay on a New Principle for Ascertaining the Curative Powers of Drugs, and Some Examinations of the Previous Principles." Cure by contraries he rejected as attacking only symptoms. He dismissed all proposed exciting, inciting, cleansing, heating, and cooling actions of medicines: these were the results not causes of alleviation. He identified the healing power of all remedies solely as their capacity to effect specific illnesses. The organism had only two possible responses to such medicines (in sequence): aggravation from the similarity, followed by stimulation of the vital force. All cures were skillful intensifications of symptoms. This was perhaps overly basic and simple, but it addressed the morass of medical contradictions.

In the same essay, Hahnemann proposed a theory of disease interaction. A severe chronic condition would, he said, prevent an acute disease of less severity from getting a hold on a system, but this was not healthy even if it reduced troublesome symptomology. An acute disease of greater severity might layer on top, and in the process "cure" a chronic disease, but the older symptoms would always return, in fact must return in any complete cure.

Hahnemann noted the partial similarity between vaccination and homeopathy; for instance, inoculation of smallpox not only protected against smallpox but often cured other diseases, including deafness, dysentery, and swollen testicles. This was not, however, a preferred solution. Indiscriminate vaccination of large populations took no account of individual defense mechanisms. Hahnemann also felt that an individual who could successfully be inoculated against a disease would likely be immune anyway or cured easily homeopathically, whereas a person responsive to the inoculation itself would develop chronic disease from the presence of this foreign substance in his system, or more precisely, its effect on his intrinsic equilibrium.

Hahnemann wrote:

> Similar symptoms in the remedy remove similar symptoms in the disease.[8]
>
> This eternal, universal law of Nature, that every disease is destroyed and cured through the similar artificial disease which the appropriate remedy has the tendency to excite, rests on the following proposition: that only one disease can exist in the body at one time, and therefore one disease must yield to the other.[9]

Hahnemann launched the science of homeopathy by testing substances on himself and recording the "artificial" diseases they induced. He preferred poisons because of their tendency to provoke a quick, discernible response. His provings of small doses of aconite, strychnine, and belladona astonished and dismayed the medical profession.

It is wrong to assume that Hahnemann fully adopted homeopathy in 1796 and never looked back. He was tentative in his reliance on new insights; for instance, he mentions, in one case of tapeworm, attempting more than sixteen allopathic medicines before, in desperation, administering white hellebore for its potential to cause a colic like the patient's. The result was such a violent colic that the person almost died, but afterward improved rapidly and permanently. From this Hahnemann was reminded not only of the power of Similars but that the artificial disease can be as dangerous as the original one.

In order to provoke a milder response, Hahnemann tried diluting his medicines even further, hoping to find the point at which they still had an effect but their aggravation was least. As expected, he found that substantial dilutions certainly caused the least aggravation, but also had the least medicinal value. Then he tried shaking the vials hard at each dilution. It is uncertain what caused him to improvise this way, and there is no explanation in Hahnemann's known writing, although many different traditionary sciences, including alchemy and Chinese medicine, urged creative or tympanic interaction with substances. Later ethnographic literature reveals that primitive peoples prepare medicines by pounding, grinding, blowing on, aiming at the Sun or stars, scraping with coral and ivory, punching once with the fist (in the case of leaves), and (in the case of pollen) suffocating a bird in the medicine before its use—all to wake the spirits in the medicine or bring spirits to attach themselves to it. African doctors have claimed that medicines contain no power in themselves but gain it solely from dynamic contact. The well-read Hahnemann may have been aware of this lore.

With his new succussed dilutions, Hahnemann took a simple step toward reducing toxicity. The results were startling, and they are still startling: the smaller the dose, not only the less the primary aggravation, but *the more profound the secondary healing*. He pursued this bizarre phenomenon to its limit.

The original homeopathic doses were at times as high as seventy grams of substance per thousand, but commonly five grams. From 1799 to 1801 Hahnemann began using notably smaller doses—1/5,000,000 of a grain of opium and 1/432,000 of a grain of dried belladona berry. During his lifetime, Hahnemann only went as far as the thirtieth centesimal ("It cannot go on to infinity," he writes,[10] but he was already at infinity, and he had opened a Pandora's box).

Rima Handley, in her biography of Hahnemann, avers that he knew exactly what he was doing:

> Hahnemann seemed to have realised that he had achieved something remarkable when he wrote in alchemical terms of the process of dilution and succussion as having liberated the "medicinal power ... from its material bonds"[11] and said that the "attenuations" were "an actual exaltation of the medicinal power, a real spiritualisation of the dynamic property, a true, astonishing unveiling and vivifying of the medicinal spirit."[12] Hahnemann undoubtably perceived that matter was being made dynamic by his preparation processes and beyond that he did not know how to continue:

> > "Now with respect to the development of physical forces from material substances by trituration, this is a very wonderful subject. It is only the ignorant vulgar that still look upon matter as dead mass, for from its interior can be elicited incredible and hitherto unsuspected powers....[13]
> > Medicinal substances are not dead masses in the ordinary sense of the term, on the contrary, their true essential nature is only dynamically spiritual ... is pure force....[14]
> > Who can say that in the millionth and billionth development the small particles of the medicinal substances have arrived at the state of atoms not susceptible to further division, of whose nature we can form not the slightest conception?"[15]

Hahnemann was reinventing Paracelsan physics.

The paradoxical increase in potency with an increase in dilution also does not occur on a linear basis or by monotonic progression. Instead there are plateaus and jumps resembling rhythmic variations, 10^{-400} being generally more powerful than 10^{-2000}, but $10^{-20,000}$ being significantly more reactive than either of these. Furthermore, overly enthusiastic repetition of homeopathic doses seems to halt activity, almost as if subtlety of transmission is necessary for homeopathic effect which too much information cancels out.[16] This could be a reason why Hahnemann accidentally discovered the quite unique "homeopathic" aspects of substance rather than another, more substantial herbal system. Homeopathy is not just cure by Similars; it is microdose isolation and amplification of certain non-pharmacological and deeply structured aspects of molecular substances applied according to the Law of Similars. These effects are apparently morphogenetic, psychosomatic, and curative without major side effects.

If such a process energizes pills, it is likely that there are ideal dilutions that respond harmonically to different planes of illness, and that continued potentization by dilution and succussion renders some medicines ineffective while empowering others. Specific potencies may also liberate subtle and unknown properties rather than confer greater absolute power.

Microdoses would one day undo homeopathy from without and within, taking the testing of remedies out of the realm of conventional chemistry and splitting Hahnemann's followers inexorably on the meanings and limits of dilutions. The mainstream criticisms of microdose were absolute and scathing right from the beginning. Dr. Hermann Schnaubert of Calila wrote satirically:

> Death has no further power over man, the homeopaths have taken away his sting! For, if shaking and rubbing a dead medicinal substance, reduced to an unimaginable size, can give an effective power passing all comprehension, surely nobody can be surprised if he sees dead men brought to life by shaking and rubbing, sustained appropriately.[17]

The paradox was intrinsic to the inability of homeopaths to place limits on degrees of dilution that were anything more than personal whims. If each dilution were, successively, more powerful, the ultimate promise and potential payoff were awesome. However, since remedies only work through the defense mechanism and the vital force, they can hardly raise the dead.

When the new fad of microdoses first arrived in America with immigrant European physicians, the full import of the system was not grasped, partly because of the foreign language of the original texts. But as the American doctors began to realize what was proposed, the response was equally derisive. In his history of American medicine, Harris Coulter notes:

> One doctor estimated that a volume of water 61 times the size of the earth was need for the 15th dilution. Others talked in terms of the Caspian or the Mediterranean, of Lake Huron or Superior.

One man calculated that 140,000 hogsheads of arsenic were dumped every year into the Ohio and Mississippi Rivers from the poisoning of rats in Pittsburgh and St. Louis, that this raised the Mississippi water to the 4th dynamization, but that it apparently had no effect on those living downstream.[18]

He quotes from two other scornful attacks:

"According to this view it is the spiritual influence of the sabre that pierces the body, not its material form. It is the spiritual influence of the club that breaks the skull. It is the spiritual influence of fried onions that causes an attack of cholera morbus."

And:

"This spiritualizing of matter by trituration is an insult to modern philosophy, and in reference to this spiritualization and tendency to mysticism, it is the mere adventitious result of habitual modes of thinking in Germany [where] science is as much pestered with spirits as poetry is."[19]

Gorman offers a contemporary version of the same skepticism:

Joel Gurin, science editor of *Consumer Reports,* a critic of homeopathy, doesn't think most people understand "the enormity" of what homeopathic theory asks one to believe. He says: "One must believe that water in some way undefined by modern science, has a memory which can be changed in a meaningful way by progressive dilution and shaking, that this 'trace resonance' in the water has a biological effect, and that all these remarkable and challenging facts were observed by a lone German physician a couple of hundred years ago. To me that's a big leap of faith."[20]

Unless one presumes that systematic succussion potentizes homeopathic microdoses, the results of homeopathic treatment have no explanation. As noted many times, homeopathy was practiced because it apparently worked, not because it could be explained. Hahnemann the doctor spawned thousands of disciples who tried his remedies with the same wonderful results; Hahnemann the philosopher and metaphysician produced only enigmas and controversies.

From 1805 until 1812, the founder lived in Torgau, near his own birthplace on the Elbe, treated patients enthusiastically, and wrote his *Organon*, the book that was to be the cornerstone of homeopathy. It was published in 1810.

Given its radical proposition, the work was reviewed generously by the medical profession, the common opinion being that the author had much of importance to say about the Law of Similars, a well-known and ancient doctrine, but tended to extend it into areas where it was inappropriate and not indicated. Doctors were smug enough not to realize that Hahnemann's attack on medicine was total, so he was viewed as an eccentric with an obsession.

Hahnemann's frustration at being, in essence, ignored, led him to return to Leipzig for a public stage, and with the paper on hellebore delivered in 1810, he won the right to lecture to medical students, as described above. In the winter term of 1812, the genius of homeopathy, fifty-seven years old and nearly bald, awkward but dressed elegantly, presented the full logos of his new-age medicine. Word spread, and the audience slowly grew. But Hahnemann was also considered an entertainment, a buffoon, with his theatrical raging, blaspheming the profession. He was belittled and quietly mocked by colleagues. It was not their acceptance he sought anymore. At the university he had acquired a group of loyal disciples from among the medical students. Hahnemann taught them to prepare their own medicines, collecting plants, minerals, insects, and the like, and doing the dilutions and succussions by hand. Together with them, he organized the first controlled provings.

Writes one:

> We lived very happily together, caring very little for the hostile glances and remarks of our colleagues. We stuck to our studies faithfully and honestly and gathered together occasionally in our teacher Hahnemann's household some time after eight in the evening.
>
> This was then the little circle formed round Hahnemann which even under the best of circumstances had to tolerate much mockery and irony and in malicious cases, hatred and persecution, not only during the student years but far beyond them. I can always remember very clearly how Hornburg was worried in his Final

Examination by the old pates and only just managed to escape being plucked, whilst miserable thickheads, not fit to wipe Hornburg's boots, passed cum laude and are now flourishing aloft here—narrow-minded but successful physicians.[21]

However, as Handley notes,

Hahnemann's stature as a practitioner now also increased as he became more practised in his new art. With the new medicine he was able successfully to treat typhoid fever, the great scourge of the time. The efficacy of homeopathy became particularly apparent in 1813, after the terrible Battle of Leipzig between the Prussian forces and Napoleon's army, retreating from the fiasco of Moscow. After three days of fighting just outside the city, there were 80,000 dead and 80,000 wounded. The streets were choked with refugees, it rained incessantly, food supplies were short and the drinking water polluted. Of the one hundred and eighty victims whom Hahnemann was able to treat, only two died. This convincing demonstration of the power of homeopathy was fully documented in Hahnemann's 1814 paper, "Treatment of Typhus Fever at Present Prevailing."[22] Hahnemann's success, however, only increased the anger of the orthodox. His flourishing practice in Leipzig also aroused opposition. For the doctors, not the least galling aspect of the new theory was the financial benefits at long last accruing to its inventor.[23]

Despite the growing popularity of the system and Hahnemann's outright fame as a healer, homeopaths never won more than temporary and conditional rights to dispense medicines in Leipzig. The local apothecaries fought to maintain their control over all pharmacy in the city, homeopathic included, though they in no way understood what was involved in preparing microdoses. Hahnemann insisted on making his own remedies because he doubted they could be made by ordinary druggists.

Handley reports that "on February 9th, 1820, Hahnemann was brought before the court and accused of encroaching upon the apothecaries' privileges by dispensing medicines. Despite his defense on March 15th, 1820, the judgment of the court was that Hahnemann was 'to cease the distributing and dispensing of any and every medicine to anybody . . . and to give no cause for severer regulations.'[24]

Without being able to prescribe and dispense, Hahnemann could not practise."[25] (The FDA holds the same potential power today over not only homeopathics but all herbal remedies, vitamins, etc.)

In 1821, Hahnemann retreated to Köthen, in Anhalt, north of Saxony, where he lived under the protection of Duke Ferdinand, whom he had treated successfully. It was hardly a haven. The gossip that preceded him warned of the arrival of an evil magician, so greeting stones were thrown through his windows. It is no wonder that Hahnemann became increasingly apocalyptic. In Köthen he wrote his last major work, *The Chronic Diseases, Their Peculiar Nature, and Their Homeopathic Cure*, which appeared in 1828. Like Freud's *Civilization and Its Discontents*, also a late book by the founder of a system, it is a pessimistic evaluation of the pathology of mankind and a concession of the mere slim possibility of any widespread or lasting cure. In a more famous document, Freud was to expose the miseries, wars, and crimes of mankind as indicators of our species' collective inability to deal with the biophysical condition of life; since civilization had suppressed mankind's true nature, psychoanalysis could offer no more than superficial relief. So with Hahnemann. Years of practice had shown him that intrinsic disease was not as curable as he once hoped, even with the Law of Similars and microdoses. He explained this persistent pathology as a collective and accumulated disease of civilization. Furthermore, he understood the failures of homeopathy to be symptoms of the underlying pathology of mankind. Early homeopaths overlooked this gloomy volume in the triumph of their own practices, but later generations have drawn its desperate conclusions. If the *Organon* is a sourcebook of practical homeopathy, *Chronic Diseases* is the bible of homeopathic esoterica.

In this oracle, Hahnemann seeks the original meaning of any disease. He defines a psora, or itch, as the primal malady, leprosy its unchecked florescence. External symptoms of itch—rashes, pimples, sores, boils—were often readily cleared up, but their internalized aggravations persisted. Deprived of its outlet on the skin, itch penetrated and weakened inner organs. Itch was also inheritable at any level to which it had been suppressed. Thus a child is born "healthy" only insofar as it has no external manifestation of civilizational disease, but it carries within it the psoric potential accumulated in the generations of its lineage.

All history is rewritten by Hahnemann as mankind's progressive internalization of surface diseases. These internalizations are potentiated as symptomatic predispositions, eventually penetrating the mental plane, from where they are exteriorized as cultural products—not only crime but art, not only plagues and insanities but philosophies and medicines. We have internalized something that was never meant to be inside us. Once there, it becomes us. Without this internalization we would not need homeopathy or any medicine. The Law of Similars and mute microdoses would radiate indiscernibly through the background of our lives.

AIDS, viewed homeopathically, is a case of an internal plague manifesting on an external plane. But it is not the plague moralists imagine, nor is its externalization a punishment for the sins they posit. The disease originated far more deeply than any transient code of behavior, perhaps even in the Stone Age, and slowly gestated.

Thus, any individual patient must be treated not only for the ailments he or she has now or those of a lifetime but for the disease level into which he or she is born. This is the scenario:

> Mankind . . . is worse off from the change in the external form of the *psora*—from leprosy down to the eruption of itch—not only because this is less visible and more secret and therefore more frequently infectious, but also because the *psora*, now mitigated externally into a mere itch, and on that account more generally spread, nevertheless still retains unchanged its original dreadful nature. Now, after being more easily repressed, the disease grows all the more unperceived within, and so, in the last three centuries, after the destruction of its chief symptom (the external skin-eruption) it plays the sad role of causing innumerable secondary symptoms; i.e., it originates a legion of chronic diseases, the source of which physicians neither surmise nor unravel, and which, therefore, they can no more cure than they could cure the original disease when accompanied by its cutaneous eruption; but these chronic diseases, as daily experience shows, were necessarily aggravated by the multitude of their faulty remedies.[26]

More practically oriented homeopaths view *The Chronic Diseases* mainly as a statement of the importance of skin ailments, their relationship to other organic and mental conditions, and the danger of repressing them. Yet Hahnemann is no mere dermatologist; he presumes himself to stand at a turning point of epochs, offering mankind its first real chance in thousands of thousands of years to break with a prehistoric scourge, driven inward and pathologized by bad medicine:

> So great a flood of numberless nervous troubles, painful ailments, spasms, ulcers (cancers), adventitious formations, dyscrasias, paralyses, consumptions and cripplings of soul, mind and body were never seen in ancient times when the *psora* mostly confined itself to its dreadful cutaneous symptom, leprosy. Only during the last few centuries has mankind been flooded with these infirmities.[27]

Hahnemann goes on to ascribe seven-eighths of all chronic diseases to suppressed psora—psora so deeply suppressed that a succession of remedies is needed to unravel the archaeology of the disease in any individual.

The other two chronic miasms, syphilis and sycosis, are relatively modern, according to Hahnemann; they emerge as complications of psora and are usually treatable with homeopathic *Mercury* and *Nitric Acid* (syphilis) and *Thuja* (sycosis). On one level syphilis and sycosis (from Greek, *sykosis*, from *sykon*, fig, not *psyche*, hence figwort disease, i.e., gonorrhea,* not psychosis) are venereal diseases. Their relationship to psora is complexly tied in with their inheritability and genital expression. They overlie psora and are the field in which it is obscured and expressed. In one sense, they are nothing more than venereal-genetic complications of basic psora. In another sense, their complexity suppresses even the natural pattern of the psora and bumps it into a more erratic vibration. While psora abounds and is infectious on an unimagined level ("the hermit on Montserrat escapes it as rarely in his rocky cell, as the little prince in his swaddling clothes of cambric"[28]), the germination of

---

* Sycosis generally describes barber's itch and scrofula, neither of which are venereal or gonorrheal. Hahnemann's special usage reveals his opinion of the source of this itch.

these other miasms requires direct genital contact or genetic transfer through offspring. They penetrate extremely deeply on emotional and spiritual planes, and their venereal symptoms can interact with prior psoric disturbances to increase pathology and provoke insanity. The psora are incurable until a successful remedy is prescribed against their overriding miasms.

Hahnemann wrote:

> Only when the whole organism feels itself transformed by this peculiar chronic-miasmatic disease, the diseased vital force endeavours to alleviate and to soothe the internal malady through the establishment of a suitable local symptom on the skin, the itch-vesicle. So long as this eruption continues in its normal form, the internal psora with its secondary ailments cannot break forth, but must remain covered, slumbering, latent and bound. While the external symptom is left in place on the skin the general health of the organism is not immediately threatened, but the illness, nevertheless, continues to grow. If the surface symptom is removed, "cured," the disease may become latent for a while, but will eventually be forced to return or seek another outlet, perhaps in a more important organ.[29]

As a book, *The Chronic Diseases* is primarily a voluminous list of psoric symptoms followed by sixteen hundred pages of antipsoric remedies and their indications. Obviously our failure to respond homeopathically to the "itch-vesicle" has led to a general deepening of pathology.

Later miasms have been announced since Hahnemann's time. Their appearance atop the previous three levels is taken as an indication of the continued deterioration of mankind. By now we must be more miasmic than human. Even our highest creations are the delusions of a terminally ill race. A current homeopathic homily claims that it was the syphilitic predisposition in Beethoven that allowed him to create beautiful music—and the syphilitic miasm in us that hears it as beautiful.

While Hahnemann's earlier writings emphasize disease as a constitutional disturbance, curable through a stimulation of the vital force by a single correct remedy in low potency, the later Hahnemann not only honored very high potencies but invented the most dilute scale in the history of physical science as celebration of them: the millesimal. This was to address the astounding depth of miasmatic illness and the degree of degradation the human race had attained by the nineteenth century.

Many homeopathic movements sprang up, not only in Leipzig where the seeds were sown, but throughout Europe and America. Hahnemann's fame spread, in part because of his successful cures during the European cholera epidemic of 1831–32. In a perception that predates microbiology, he describes certain minute but discrete disease entities. He names the "cholera miasm" an "organism of lower order" and later speaks of an "invisible cloud of perhaps millions of such miasmatic living organisms, which, first brought to life on the broad and marshy shores of the tepid Ganges, are continually seeking out man to his destruction."[30]

His researches had carried him well past the original proposition, but when he came down, like Moses from the mountain, he found his disciples worshipping the idols. He too cracked the tablets of God. Homeopathy survived the split for a long time, but eventually it proved fatal.

Hahnemann wrote angrily in a newspaper:

I have heard for a long time and with displeasure, that some in Leipsic, who pretend to be Homeopaths, allow their patients to choose whether they shall be treated homeopathically or allopathically ... let them ... not require of me that I should recognize them as my true disciples. ...

Blood-letting, the application of leeches and Spanish flies, the use of fontanels and setons, mustard plasters and medicated bags, embrocations with salves and aromatic spirits, emetics, purgatives, various sorts of warm baths, pernicious doses of calomel, quinine, opium and musk, are some of the quackeries by which, when used in conjunction with homeopathic prescriptions, we are able to recognize the crypto-homeopath, trying to make himself popular. ... They swagger in the cradle of homeopathic science (as they choose to call Leipsic) where its founder first stepped forward as a teacher. But behold! I have never yet acknowledged you; away from me, ye medical —![31] [The newspaper chose not to print the word.]

In the last years of his life, Hahnemann renounced many doctors and hospitals he had initially blessed or helped found. As his fame spread, he charged outrageous sums of money for his services while continuing to work in isolation on later editions of the *Organon*. He was already surrounded with controversy and myth when a singular and unexpected event whisked him away from his disciples and practice.

Hahnemann's wife of forty-nine years died in the spring of 1830, and in 1834, a French woman, thirty-two years of age, having been inspired by the *Organon*, arrived in Köthen, ostensibly to meet the author in person and seek his aid.

> It is clear that what started out as a professional consultation soon took an unforeseen turn. Within three days of their meeting Hahnemann had proposed to Mélanie, and she had accepted. She had at last found a man she could admire as well as love, and he found himself kissing and embracing her in not quite the "paternal" manner he had originally intended. Over the following three months Mélanie wrote a number of letters to him[31] which show how immediate and powerful was the attraction between them. In only her second letter she wrote: "You have told me: 'I have never loved anyone so much as you, we shall love each other till eternity.' You have said: 'I cannot live any longer without you, stay with me for ever; we must be married.'" She had responded: "I can no longer live now without your good opinion and love;" and "you will always be my husband in my thoughts; no other man will ever lay a profane hand on me, no mouth other than yours will kiss my mouth. I give you my faith, and I swear to you eternal love and fidelity."[32]

They were married in June of 1835. He was eighty. He had always praised and even prescribed marriage, on one occasion just before remarrying calling it "a general specific for body and soul."[33]

With Marie Mélanie Hahnemann, he moved to Paris, where she presented him to the French homeopathic community. It was as though, on a journey to the land of the dead, she had recovered Hippocrates himself.

Hahnemann lived in Paris until his eighty-ninth year, practicing medicine, continuing his revisions of his books, and preaching against the ravages of allopathy and the half-breeds. He was cared for, admired, and pampered there. The controversy that surrounded his departure from Leipzig, however, grew in his absence. Reports from Paris indicated that his wife had taken over his practice, that no one could see Hahnemann except through her, and that she alone did the diagnosis and prescribing while he sat, impassive and observing. It is also reported that he prescribed two remedies at one time, a shocking violation of the single cure. In any case, the combination of his charisma and medical fame as a miracle physician and the notoriety of his marriage to a woman well-known in French intellectual and artistic circles brought no end of wealthy and notable patients and curiosity-seekers to the Hahnemanns' door.

Apparently, Madame Hahnemann did take over her husband's practice, but no easy conclusion can be drawn from this, and certainly not that the old man was bewitched and corrupted by her. He chose this particular form of retirement and discipleship through her. Perhaps he saw in her a strength, for she did later become a homeopathic physician of renown and talent.

She was certainly aware of the delicacy of the situation. Early on she wrote of Hahnemann's daughters: "They treat me like an adventuress who has probably come to seduce you, and you (the author of the *Organon*) like a feeble and libertine old man."[34]

From his Paris outpost, Hahnemann was also able to aid the spread and advancement of homeopathy. His instruction of an English physician from India led to the founding of a separate homeopathic tradition on the subcontinent. If this was a decline or senility, it was an energetic one.

Hahnemann also dropped out of touch with former associates and abandoned his children in Saxony, even in his will. His death, on July 2, 1843, went unannounced for many weeks, and his burial was private, unknown to friends and family, either in France or Saxony. Marie Mélanie Hahnemann buried her husband above the two other spouses she had already outlived by the age of thirty-two, at the same grave site—and she kept the sixth revision of the *Organon* unavailable during her lifetime, likely because its requirements for publication overwhelmed her.

Hahnemann was, all his life, a puritanical Christian, even in his quite exuberant departures from the usual limitation of that persuasion. Obsessed with keeping himself healthy, he punctuated his scholarship with regular exercise. He was a stern father, unyielding teacher and master—and absolutely blind to any other psychological or spiritual system. He had the kind of mind and attention that bores to the center of things, through all diversions and distractions. But he never turned that analysis back on his own condition, either his psychospiritual condition or the unexamined research from which he formed his theories. He was a mystic by ideology only.

So homeopathy comes to us from Hahnemann as a system of concrete epigrams trapped in a spiritual cosmology. There are plants, animals, minerals, flesh-and-blood people, pathologies; beneath is a pattern of universal oscillations and energies. Hahnemann's original loyalty may have been to physical science, botany, and industrial chemistry, but by the time the system was completed and he was an old man, spirit had totally replaced matter. It was Hahnemann's Puritanical stubbornness that led him to keep calling this mishmash regular old medicine and science, and to attempt to deliver it to the world as that—a stubbornness that also made the clinical practice of magic possible. Even today, as William Blake pronounced, physics too is a dream from which we have yet to awake.

The only way back into matter for Hahnemann would have been through mind, but he never admitted mind either as psyche or episteme into his system, hence homeopathy has a nonintersecting, parallel course with psychiatry. Jung later induced spirit back into matter through layers of personal and collective psyche. The marriage yielded geometric shapes, laws of science, myths, etc., simultaneously in flowers, starfish, and galaxies, as we saw in Whitmont's interpretations in the last chapter. The "archetypes" are the mind behind matter which mind in matter recognizes in itself and all things.

Hahnemann's "archetypes" were instead imprinted on balls of milk sugar and alcohol—each ball chemically inert, but each containing a universe to be manifested through a living system. By ignoring mind, Hahnemann was forced to find intelligence behind matter. The homeopathic medicines *are* the Jungian archetypes in hologrammatic form.

In the end, it would appear, the undiagnosed spirituality of Hahnemann's life ran riot. His rigid judgmentalism condemned mankind to chronic diseases and sabotaged the very movement he had spawned. At the same time, he fell before the attractions of the anima and was lured from family and disciples into a foreign country by a pixie skilled in such escapades, who withheld his final work and buried him unnamed in a tomb with her earlier lovers.

Yet this last escapade was a heroic statement of homeopathic vitality, to adventure amorously rather than to stay in Leipzig and squabble until death. One Saxon journalist accused him of trying "to prove to the world how his system has been glorified in him.... The young man is still vigorous and strong, and challenges all Allopaths: imitate me if you can!"[35] Hahnemann had long ago cast his lot in strange lands with unknown voices, and in his eighties, with his scholarship completed, he vanished into exile again.

The system already a mongrel, he returned to the pagan forces he never acknowledged or bowed to but whose offspring it was. Homeopathy had been his destiny and reigning achievement, but it took him a lifetime to get there, and then transform it back into a mystery: one remedy, many remedies; material medicine, spiritual medicine; visible disease, hidden disease; curable ailments, submerged miasmatic complexes. No wonder homeopathy has sought a founder and a clarification ever since.

Chapter 5

The Homeopathic Tradition in America

During the nineteenth century the American allopathic profession was simply one of many healing modalities. Midwives, Indian doctors, and lay herbal practitioners thrived; native manipulative systems such as osteopathy and chiropractic spread through their own medical colleges. Homeopathy likewise built its own academy. Alternative medicine today is in fact a fulfillment and florescence of an original multicultural diversity.

North American naturopathy was a blend of traditional European botanicals with remedies developed in the New World. These indigenous pharmacies had been tested for generations, and they were liberally incorporated by the newcomers. A steam bath and herbal treatment of the New Hampshire farmer Samuel Thomson was immensely popular, and his followers, operating their own hospitals, drug manufacturing houses, and drugstores, had an astonishing three million adherents in 1839 when the whole population of the United States was estimated to be seventeen million.

Meanwhile, the system of "irritable mechanism," developed by Cullen and John Brown in England, was the fashion in allopathic American medicine. The body was portrayed as a machine made out of flesh, with membranous pipes, pulleys, levers, and strainers, its hydraulics maintained by the breath and the heart. Medicines were prescribed either to provoke or relax spasms. For an overactive system, vomiting was induced or blood drawn off and cold baths administered. Even though bleeding was a relaxant, some doctors bled to stimulate, with an epicyclic image to explain the contradictory effect. Opium, liquors, hot baths, garlic, mercury, and wine by the gallon were used as stimulants for phlegmatic ailments. This theory lingers even today in the laxatives that "break up" stalled matter in the bowels, the magnesias, milks, and vegetable antacids given for an overactive stomach, and even, in a sense, the antibiotics that attack bacteria. Any trip to a drugstore shows the enormity of our commitment to a mechanical attack on our pain.

Eighteenth-century oversimplification, reinforced by fad, had settled on one mercurous chloride medicine, originally a stimulant, as the absolute cure-all. Called "calomel," after the Greek for "beautiful black," though its final form was a white powder, it was used in high doses for every imaginable illness and as a general preventative for future ailments. Benjamin Rush, the most respected American physician of the late eighteenth and early nineteenth centuries, was a strong advocate of mercury and bloodletting. Coulter describes a scene from the 1793 yellow fever epidemic in Philadelphia:

> Rush was surrounded one day . . . by a crowd in Kensington, north of Philadelphia. All implored him to come and treat their families.
> There were several hundred. Rush, without stepping down, threw back the top of his curricle, and addressed the multitude "with a few conciliatory remarks." Then he cried in a loud voice, "I treat my patients successfully by bloodletting and copious purging with calomel and jalap—and I advise you, my good friends, to use the same remedies."
> "What?" called a voice from the crowd, "bleed and purge every one?"
> "Yes!" said the doctor. "Bleed and purge all Kensington! Drive on, Ben!"[1]

Many people suffered from undiagnosed chronic disease caused by calomel; mercury poisoning was common during this era. Intuiting this, mothers often clutched their children in the presence of the doctor and would not let them be treated, despite malaria, croup, and other serious respiratory and intestinal diseases.

Most historians of medicine claim that the early American homeopaths encountered a corrupt, out-of-control profession and then exploited people's fear and anger. They were successful merely because they did not use mercury or draw blood. They had the uncanny luck to encounter a situation in which they could be heroes by prescribing "nothing." If homeopaths had been giving placebos only, as these historians assert, they still would have been doing more good than most calomel and bloodletting hacks. This is allopathy's current explanation for homeopathy's early popularity, for modern allopathy has no more use for Rush's medicine than homeopaths did.

When homeopathy arrived in America, the medical mainstream did not have a clear sense of what it was. Some assumed it was just orthodox German medicine, and they accepted it. Others lumped it together with Indian medicine and Thomsonian treatment as another botanical. It was generally considered a viable though specialized form of healing in no way in conflict with allopathy.

The first homeopaths began to practice in the United States in the mid-1820s. Most were immigrant doctors, but a few American-born physicians learned the system by correspondence, or visits to Europe. A graduate of Wurtzburg University, Constantine Hering founded the first American school of homeopathy, the Nordamerikanisch Akademie der Homeopathischen Heilkunst, in Allentown, Pennsylvania, in 1835, with instruction in German. It lasted six years, and seven years after its closing, he replaced it with the Homeopathic Medical College in Philadelphia. Students from this college practiced primarily in the Middle Atlantic and southern states, while fresh homeopaths from Germany took on clientele on the East Coast and throughout the Midwest. As early as 1844, three years before the establishment of the AMA, the American Institute of Homeopathy was founded in order to license their own physicians and maintain standards of practice. This body also served as a clearing-house for the provings of North American native plants and other new remedies. The AMA was later formed in reaction to the homeopaths as a business guild, to protect the interests of its physicians. It was never a neutral scientific body.

As homeopathic works were translated into English and homeopathic doctors became more ubiquitous, the allopaths began to realize this was not just another branch of their own science; it was a threat to their very existence, for it proposed to supersede them with a superior system.

Homeopathy soon became the prince of the medical underground. It appealed to the already vast audience of the naturopaths and Thomsonians, yet provided parents with authoritative doctors trained in medical schools who gave pleasant-tasting sugar pills (in contrast to the high doses of foul-tasting mercury). They heard out one's full symptoms and life history and were knowledgeable without being condescending.

Professional medicine initially reacted by denouncing homeopathy as a European scam intended to hoodwink backwoods Americans. "Sane men," doctors said, "could hardly be fooled by such patent foolishness."

This was a transitional time in America, marked by a continuing border war between Missouri and Kansas, the invention of daytime bank and train robberies by Confederate raiders Frank and Jesse James, coal mine strikes in Idaho (where anarchist miners dynamited trainloads of scabs, their own mines, plus the Governor himself); exotic religious cults and epiphanies sprang up weekly.

Another reason for the increasing popularity of homeopathy was the outward simplicity of the system. A lay practitioner need know nothing about physiology or chemistry; it is a matter of matching actual symptoms against lists in a repertory. The pills could be dispensed by clergymen, lawyers, and housewives. Hering himself put out a kit for simple and common maladies, with complete instructions; the pills were identified only by numbers. A certain condition might require number 8, but if the fever was higher, number 3 was used, number 12 if the ailment was primarily on the right side, number 18 if it turned into a rash. It was not uncommon for the wives and children of allopaths to treat their families secretly in this way while the sire failed even to notice. The stern decrees of Hahnemann had become an American parlor game. Yet it freed people from staggering medical bills and from a terror of medicine that existed in the nineteenth century.

Its entire theory of anatomy and irritability at stake, allopathy rebelled with scathing critiques.

Wrote one doctor: "[The] whole art is reduced to the precision of a game of ninepins."[2]

Another: "The entire range of diseases, the entire range of therapeutics, converted into Chinese puzzles; the phenomena of diseases and the effects of drugs upon them treated as algebraical equations."[3]

These were legitimate doubts.

Though the serious weaknesses in homeopathy were being exposed, homeopaths generally ignored them. They were at the height of their success through the 1870s and 1880s, doing three to seven times the business of allopaths, with the editorial support of the *Detroit Daily Tribune* and *The New York Times* behind them, the backing of politicians and business interests, and a lobby much like today's gun lobby in the Republican Party. During the yellow fever epidemic of the 1870s in the South, homeopaths not only used their microdoses successfully, but succeeded in legislating sanitary reforms in the canals, sewage systems, dry wells, and bogs around Savannah and New Orleans. Elsewhere, homeopaths were appointed to state medical boards and federal pension examination boards. They were supported by government funds and covered by insurance companies. There were hundreds of homeopathic hospitals, clinics, insane asylums, nursing homes, orphanages, and schools in the United States.

The first shot was actually fired in 1842 when the New York State Medical Society ruled that homeopathy was a form of quackery, not science, and "a departure from the principles of a well defined system of medical ethics."[4] Committee members argued that homeopathy should *not* be granted immunity as another medical system with its own licensing because it dealt in pretentiously named vacuous sugar tablets under the guise of pharmacy. Four years later, when the National Medical Convention met in New York to review the problem, the members concluded that the success of homeopathy must be a result of their own bad marketing and public relations, for homeopathic pills were placebos only. Since many of their own medical schools gave bogus degrees and it was often impossible to tell the difference between a pseudomedical college and a legitimate training program, they decided first to police their own ranks. If they could define who they were and isolate the rest as quacks, then homeopaths could be kicked out with the other medical illusionists. Their publicized long-term goal was the improvement of medical education, but their true short-term goal was the ostracism of the homeopaths. This led to the debut of the American Medical Association.

In its charter, the AMA withheld membership from state and local medical organizations unless they assured the national organization that no homeopaths belonged. Only Massachusetts balked. In 1856 the AMA banned any discussion of homeopathic medical theory in its journals and threatened the expulsion of any doctor who consulted with a homeopath. Allopaths married to homeopaths were also expelled.

The AMA has historically argued that its stance was against all quackery, in an attempt to professionalize the medical occupation. Documents make it clear, though, that homeopathy was the prime target. With their own medical societies, journals, and courses in the medical schools, homeopaths were the sole serious academic competitors.

Initially, the strategy failed. Most people viewed medical philosophy as an esoteric issue and called on their favorite local physicians regardless of affinity. Doctors were also used to cooperating with each other and taking each others' patients in emergencies. The public was generally offended by a new rule that seemed arbitrary and excluded cherished doctors, in fact sometimes the only doctor in a region. It seemed more like politics than medicine. The moral authority of the AMA today is a relatively recent event.

Many medical schools did bow, however, to the tightened regime, though some, the University of Michigan in particular, retained a homeopathic curriculum and forced their own compromise on the AMA. In Michigan, many members of the Board of Regents were patients of homeopaths, and elected officials were more inclined to favor homeopathy than the AMA.

Most significant, ultimately, was the inevitable merger of the two systems. The average homeopath, as we pointed out, already practiced allopathy too, as part of a general "new" medicine. Innovative procedures were, in a sense, nondenominational, adopted by everyone. Even as homeopathy survived the frontal attack, the number of pure traditional homeopaths sharply declined.

If allopaths did not learn to give spiritual doses, they gradually came to the conclusion that their own heroic doses were extreme and that sheer mass of medicine did not equal amount of healing. Professional acceptance of specifics returned, and the standard medicine chest was remodeled. Calomel, quinine, and jalap passed out of fashion and, with them, bleeding. Doctors experimented with different natural remedies and compounds innovated by the drug companies. Even if a doctor did not accept homeopathic microdose, he could prescribe the same substance in material form. If he liked the medicine but not the Law of Similars, he could explain its action mechanically, e.g., that *Kali Nitricum*, or St. Ignatius' Bean, had the power to stimulate the system. Since much of homeopathic pharmacy came from Classic, Mediaeval, and Arabic sources, allopathic pharmacy was also returning to its own origin in adopting homeopathically prepared substances. It was not hard for homeopaths to abandon their purity and join the stampede.

The earlier cholera epidemic of 1849 had an enormous impact in promoting medical change. The medical establishment admitted freely that it had no cure for this condition. Hahnemann had used *Camphor* early in the disease for its similar alternating diarrhea and constipation. The American school tried this remedy with success. In Cincinnati, homeopaths claimed a 97 percent cure rate in over a thousand cases and published a daily list of their patients in the newspaper, giving the names and addresses of those who were cured and those who died. Bleeding was of little use, though it remained the allopathic standby.

Nonhomeopathic doctors had a hard time believing the *Camphor* results. Elaborate explanatory hypotheses for homeopathic cures were concocted: late-acting allopathic remedies, hypnotism, and power of suggestion (or even the wrongness of their own techniques, hence the advantage of no treatment at all). Perhaps the most common interpretation was that the unusually high cure rate of the homeopaths came not from their medicines but their rules of hygiene and diet. This belief literally changed allopathy from within, without turning it quite into homeopathy. So both systems approached each other without most doctors realizing the contradictions in basic theory. The AMA never had to defeat homeopathy. Allopathy became palatable enough for many homeopaths. Likewise, some allopaths found advantages in Similars.

One prominent allopath, William Holcombe, wrote of his guilt and sleeplessness the day he administered his first homeopathic remedies out of frustration with nothing else working:

> The spirit of Allopathy, terrible as a nightmare, came down fiercely upon me and would not let me rest. What right had I to dose that poor fellow with Hahnemann's medicinal moonshine?[5]

Nowadays people shrug and smile if one suggests that homeopathy ever represented enough of a threat to bring the powerful AMA into being. How quickly whole stages of history disappear! Major institutions collapse, and the next generation is born into a different world. The remains of the old homeopathic "empire" are scattered throughout the United States, especially in the eastern half, like the Southern Cult of pre-Columbian Indians. The hospitals and other buildings (and even Hahnemann's name) have been taken over by other parties. Parts of libraries were moved out of the science section into storage facilities or sold at a quarter a volume. (In 1968 I found a wealth of homeopathy books in a remote corner of the University of Michigan Medical Library. No doubt, with dramatically growing interest in homeopathy, these have since gone the way of the alchemy collections in the same library: the rare-book room for those not already stolen. New, young homeopaths have "liberated" such volumes for years from various collections on the grounds that they were "political-industrial prisoners," as one gung-ho convert told me.)

Nineteenth-century homeopathy is a mere blink of the eye away. It is fading names on buildings, chiseled in stone and then covered by a temporary wooden sign announcing a new clinic or a multimillion-dollar health facility. The former patients are, if still alive, in their seventies and eighties. They patronized the last of the old-breed doctors, until these also died, with no one to take over their practices.

It is difficult to believe that something so fervent ended so abruptly or started up again so powerfully.

Traditional homeopathy, in fact, was doomed to failure from the beginning. It was an uncompromising, rigid system, demanding a commitment and purism few could maintain, especially in light of very sane demonstrations that the whole premise was unscientific. Hahnemann demanded strict adherence to the Law of Similars to find the correct remedy; there was no leeway on this. Either one was discerning enough to work through the symptoms and come to a clear picture of the disease or one was not.

A few of Hahnemann's early students were purists, but most later practitioners used homeopathy as simply another tool. If homeopathic procedure failed, there were many other systems of medicine to fall back on, including treatment by opposites. Hahnemann once upon a time viewed these hybrids as "worse than allopaths . . . amphibians . . . still creeping in the mud of the allopathic marsh . . . who only rarely venture to raise their heads in freedom toward the ethereal truth."[6]

After all, if doctors felt there was an alternative to the strict delayering of disease, they would never follow their cases through to the psoric base and homeopathy itself would be faulted for their inability to produce a lasting cure. Furthermore, it made little sense first to heighten and then to reduce the same symptoms and call each an attempt at cure.

Many homeopaths, however, took the liberal position: the Law of Similars was just one law of nature and should be used along with other laws. They preferred low potencies because these still had some physical substance in them and were compatible with overall American pharmacy. For the pure Hahnemannians, however, the high potencies were the most effective tool for getting at deep-seated disease and made up the core of their practice. The argument of their colleagues against nonmaterial doses was, after all, nothing more than the identical argument allopaths had used against homeopathy from the beginning.

At this point, too, the ranks of homeopathy swelled with newcomers and converts from the yellow fever and cholera epidemic days. These doctors were poorly trained in the repertory and materia medica and probably still practiced allopathy if with a homeopathic bent. They were attempting to follow the current and would likewise be swept along with it into general medicine.

Homeopathic literature reflected the change in attitude. Homeopaths themselves heralded the new scientific knowledge about pathology as a basis for genuinely informed prescription and regarded the days when they had to rely only on the totality of symptoms as a kind of dark age, a groping in the dark. They developed a new language of "important symptoms" and streamlined the repertory, giving all the remedies an active, almost Solidist explanation.

The cultural basis for each medicine's popularity cannot be underestimated. Homeopathy was buoyed by the basic life-style of the mid-nineteenth century, but allopathy benefited from twentieth-century demographic shifts. Specialization became as popular and necessary in medicine as in other areas of industrial society, and suddenly the homeopathic general practitioners seemed as old-fashioned as they had once seemed modern. Their books became outdated; they were isolated from general science. At one point, they caused less pain than the allopaths, but with better palliative and first-aid drugs, allopathy had at least drawn even—and without the patient having to suffer a period of trial and error and ensuing aggravation.

Initially homeopathy was less expensive, but that changed too. A homeopath needed more time with his patients, so he charged a high sum for the first case-taking visit. That was not a drawback when allopaths used their own expensive treatments. Now suddenly the family homeopath was in competition with cut-rate medicine. He had also been used to continued contact with not only single patients but families over generations. That continuity supported his detailed and accurate symptom-assessment and ensured a stable clientele. However, after the transportation revolution of the late nineteenth and early twentieth centuries, that clientele began to fission. People could not move their medical philosophies across the country, so they came to count on standardization from locale to locale. A shifting populace led to quick prescribing and encouraged the most expedient in both allopathy and homeopathy. Trapped by economic and social forces beyond their control, many homeopaths resorted to any medicines that would get quick results.

The most orthodox group of Hahnemannians, who represented the power within the professional organizations, were fundamentalists, with the *Organon* as their Bible. They continued to use Hahnemann's miasmatic symptomology even after it became dated and less applicable diagnostically. The style of the *Organon* became required, perhaps not in place of its substance but as well as its substance. They forgot that Hahnemann had written in the language of his day, adapting his own contemporary disease terms to explain unknown disease processes.

As long as homeopathic philosophy opposed the very notion that a disease could be known, it opposed rationalist science. Hahnemannian homeopathy became a religion—a laboratory branch of spiritualism. For the believer, research into disease cause was equated with biblically forbidden research into the evolution of man, the genesis of life. Adam's inquiry was original sin with a psoric impulse at its base. The disease cause was unknown because it was meant to be unknowable. Too much was already made of the obvious affinity of the miasms with "unclean sexuality" for homeopathy ever to have any claim at being socially progressive or philosophically objective.

Homeopathic purists were like church fathers from the Old Country who stood against the presumed radical excesses of secularization and democracy and who had no sympathy for difficulties a young doctor faced in trying to survive economically. They may have been resourceful case-takers, but they were not tolerant elders. Bewitched by their own rigidity and antimodernism, they missed the point of the *fin de siècle* paradigm shift.

They attacked modern science as if it were uniform and atheistic, but their perspective was Hahnemann's eighteenth-century German theism. Homeopathy, or at least Hahnemannian homeopathy, could have benefited from a branch of science that was to discover untold, greater quantum fractal mysteries in nature and that was to unleash a more powerful and generous God at the base of matter. This science in fact would one day rediscover homeopathy. Instead, Hahnemann was canonized and homeopathy bowed out on the side of literalism, even though the microdose principle and the theory of miasms could not be applied literally.

Purism was a strategic error, but it was unavoidable. The *Organon* suggested a deeper dialectic, but it did not honor it. Hahnemann's personality may have contained seeds of an ultimate transformative genius, but he was careful to check any revolutionary tendency except for the occasional rages and a seeming last apostasy.

As against a medicine of unnecessary bloodletting and general poisoning, homeopathy was an angel and guardian of the sick. When the issues became more subtle and the gap between purisms greater, orthodox homeopathy resorted, unaware, to rhetoric and dogma. Sloppy homeopathy was no better, for it resorted to the unexamined jargon of progressive liberal science. In so doing, it abandoned the principle that alone made homeopathy distinct. Overall, homeopathy lost its social context on one side and its scientific credentials on the other. It alienated all its potential twentieth-century constituencies.

From this point on, there were individual gifted practitioners, but professional homeopathy was doomed. Only the purists could maintain the science, and only the "half-breeds" could maintain cultural relevance.

Born on the other side of this divide (with two World Wars and the full transmutation of the twentieth century in the middle), we often miss the impact of what happened. When we "rediscover" pure homeopathy, we assume that its principles have always been consistent and ideologically neutral. We imagine its relationship to scientific inquiry along only one order of complication. A combination of Vitalism and superstitious literalism is confusing to us. Our global, multicultural tolerance allows a spiritual synthesis far beyond the imagination of nineteenth-century physicians on all sides of the argument. We have lived long enough past Newton, Darwin, and Cullen to realize the truth in each of their works, while excusing gaps and "errors." In the nineteenth century, the purists of all ilk stuck to their fundamentalisms and did not imagine that anything would survive atheistic science, let alone God. Their God (or their modernistic atheism), however, was as much a cultural artifact as their science. A larger "process" deity has since emerged from the tumult. We are free to practice homeopathy on a "patent pending" basis and to improvise our belief system from day to day. Einstein and Heisenberg have dislodged and potentiated our entire belief quotient, they as well as Gertrude Stein and Paul Klee. The "half-breeds" had no such way to stick to homeopathic principle and also participate in new science, so they were eventually absorbed into allopathy, priests who forgot their own ceremonies.

The purists went down a different road of extinction; they maintained Hahnemann's dated politics, allying themselves with conservative positions in American thought, often taking racist and ultracapitalist positions that reflected more the cultural conventions of Hahnemann's time than their own world. Homeopathy, as a system of thought, unfortunately, became identified with these positions. Radical, or for that matter mainstream, progressive ideas were slandered as "disease complexes" by strict homeopaths. Psychoanalysis and social work were mocked and dismissed. One homeopathic journal of the late 1960s departed from medical issues only to urge a return to Christ and the immediate bombing of Hanoi. It is all the more ironic that homeopathy was finally rescued by post-Einsteinian scientists and the radical counterculture. But it was rescued in a way that totally changed its social context while maintaining original Hahnemannian principles.

Reborn homeopathy is more sophisticated and refined than its forebear as well as more integrated into other holistic disciplines. Now that practitioners generally accept (even if they do not fully understand) that microdoses do not and cannot work according to a standard allopathic paradigm, they are free to move outside traditional homeopathic literalism and begin to explore actual efficacies and inefficacies. They also have no stake in the old battles. They gain exactly the credibility for challenging scientistic arrogance and technological hegemony their predecessors feared losing a century ago in abandoning the scientific revolution.

A dramatic pharmaceutical revolution played a role in the transformation of all medicine. When the unpopular calomel-style drugs passed into disuse, they were replaced by a mixture of American Indian medicines, substances originating in homeopathy, and new laboratory compounds. Coulter's survey of contemporary medicines derived from homeopathy during the late nineteenth century includes *Hellebore, Bryonia, Cactus* (as a heart medicine), *Poison Ivy* (homeopathic *Rhus Toxicodendron*), *Cocculus Indicus, Drosera Rotundifolia* (for whooping cough), *Cannabis* (for gonorrhea), *Pulsatilla Nigricans, Conium* (for cancer and paralysis), and *Apis Mellifica* (bee poison for rheumatism).[7]

The common use of other medicines was extended by homeopathic proving. Camphor for cholera is one example. Homeopathy also introduced the use of *Thuja Occidentalis* (the Arbor Vitae) for secondary illness caused by vaccination and gonorrhea. Poison Nut and Red Pepper came to be prescribed in paralysis and hemorrhoids, respectively; *Ailanthus Glandulosa* for scarlet fever and Coffee for headaches were also homeopathic extensions.[8] They, along with all the other indigenous herbal medicines, are lost in the synthetic mêlée of modern pharmacy, but they lie at its base along with medicines of the rainforest and outback introduced more recently. At one point, the newly powerful drug factories appeared poised to take over the field of healing and render all doctors obsolete. Coulter writes:

> Sharpe and Dohme, E. R. Squibb, and Frederick Stearns got their start during the Civil War and were later joined by William R. Warner (1866), Parke-Davis (1867), Mallinckrodt Chemica Works (1867), Eli Lilly (1876), William S. Merrell, H. M. Merrell, E. Merck, Abbott Laboratories, and others. For the first decade these firms competed in terms of the traditional medicines used by the profession. In the 1870s, however, it became clear that this was too narrow a channel for disposing of the production of an ever-growing industry, and the outcome was an invasion by these "ethical" drug companies of the patent-medicine field.[9]

That is, drug companies changed from the production of simple medicines whose ingredients were familiar to physicians and whose uses were established by tradition to the invention and marketing of new synthetic compounds, whose basic chemistry was unknown by doctors and whose uses had to be determined by chemical-mechanical research. These new medicines were known as "proprietaries." Their ingredients were the trade secrets of the drug companies producing them, and their application was no more than a designation on the label. These could be marketed directly through the pharmacies to the clients, who would be "informed" by advertising rather than medical prescription. Even if a doctor were to intercede between the drug company and the pharmacy, he would be as ignorant as the patient, since he did not know either the make-up or effects of the compounds.

The AMA was wary and critical from the beginning:

> The first stupendous error, one which is so vast in its influence that it hangs like a withering blight over the individuality of every man in the profession, is the dictation of innumerable pharmaceutical companies, the self-constituted advisers in the treatment of diseases about which they know nothing, to the entire profession. . . . They are so solicitous that they flood your office with blatant literature, full of bombastic claims and cure-alls, and I am sorry to say, too frequently with certificates or articles used by permission from physicians who call themselves reputable.[10]

In 1900 the American medical profession was at war with every system that threatened it, and Squibb, Parke-Davis, et al., were as much threats as the disciples of Hahnemann. The moment of conflict was disingenuously seized by both industries. The drug companies and doctors suddenly recognized each other as allies, sensing, perhaps always, that the homeopaths were their common enemy, in terms of both medical-chemical principle and commercial ethics. They then collaborated in the sort of "public be damned" conspiracy of silence that has become the hallmark of an age of amoral corporations ever since. They will do it again, under new names, every time they feel they have to.

Parke-Davis and Squibb began publishing their own medical literature. Never openly propagandist, seemingly historical and scientific in intent, their pamphlets and periodicals rewrote history in favor of the proprietary medicines, congratulating the medical profession for being in the vanguard of new science.

Parke-Davis alone was responsible for a startling number of "respectable" medical journals: *New Preparations, Detroit Medical Journal, American Lancet, Therapeutic Gazette, Medical Age, Druggists' Bulletin,* and *Medicine.*[11] In some cases, they purchased existing journals and renamed them; in other cases, they expanded house organs into so-called scientific publications, with the addition to their staff of professors of medicine and well-known doctors. Many physicians advanced professionally mainly by their association with the journals.

But patronage did not stop with the direct issuing of publications. Virtually all other medical journals, at least all the major ones, including the *Journal of the American Medical Association (JAMA)*, were supported through the advertising of proprietary medicines. Doctors were solicited as successfully as the public had been. And the journals, which gave the drug manufacturers their necessary legitimacy, at the same time anointed the AMA from the status of another political party to a scientific and professional body representing the whole medical profession. Gradually, the resistance to proprietary medicines quieted, and the drug companies, under protection of the secrecy of their products in a market economy, were held only to the most perfunctory disclosure of the contents of drugs advertised in medical journals.

Medicine gradually synergized. A phase came in which both allopathy and homeopathy disappeared into archaisms. A new system arose, with controlled experiments, advanced machinery, modern facilities, and a microbiological pharmacy. A fellowship of science was proclaimed: "We are all now professionals," the argument went. "No more schools and sectarian positions, only general universal objective medicine." It was a compelling argument. But since homeopathic and allopathic principles are opposed, the new system had to work by one principle rather than another, and it was predominantly allopathic in its allegiance.

From 1899 to 1911 George H. Simmons was general secretary of the American Medical Association and editor of the *JAMA*. He remained editor until 1924. Notably, he was once a homeopath (in Nebraska), and, according to Coulter, an ardent one. After his conversion to allopathy, he was well qualified to handle the thorny issue. Instead of continuing the long-standing attack, he went against precedent (and against much of the AMA membership) in welcoming not only homeopaths but all alternative practitioners into the AMA (as long as the former stopped calling themselves "homeopaths" and stopped using homeopathic medicines). They were invited in celebration of the end of sectarianism. A great number of homeopaths accepted, especially low-potency practitioners, who felt more cut off from their fault-finding Hahnemannian brethren than their mainstream opponents. Homeopathic pharmacies became standard American drugstores, carrying proprietaries and patent medicines because the public, as usual uninvolved in the philosophical issues, demanded them. These drugs were widely advertised and prescribed. The stores also continued to carry homeopathic remedies until they were no longer in demand.

The continued passage of so many homeopathic doctors into general nonhomeopathic practice severely weakened the homeopathic movement. Mainstream allopathy constantly advanced the position that the aim of medicine was to effect cures of the sick and not to hold to any rigid positions at the expense of that. The *JAMA* declared:

> It is a favorable sign to find a faithful follower of Hahnemann who acknowledges the natural tendency of which most medical men are aware, and it causes us to renew our hope that the time is not so very distant when the believers in the efficacy of dilutions will cease to shut themselves up in a "school" and will become a part of the regular medical profession, the members of which are ready and anxious to employ any and every means which can be scientifically shown to have a favorable influence upon the course of disease.[12]

The American Institute of Homeopathy began a countermovement in 1910, but individual homeopaths were not interested in anything that smacked of either unionism or hucksterism. They guarded their practices like hawks, not necessarily training any disciples to replace them. When the last generation of homeopathic doctors died out, the practice died with them. Even the homeopathic medical schools were conveniently converted to allopathy, with elective courses in homeopathy. No one wanted to waste a working facility. The lower-potency prescribers, of course, felt quite at home with courses in anatomy, physiology, and pathology. Those who taught materia medica were kept on in acknowledgment of the school charters but were regarded as relics, "historians" of medicine. This embarrassment proved that Hahnemann was right when he denied the possibility of half-homeopathy. Half-homeopathy is nonhomeopathy.

The field secretary hired by the American Institute of Homeopathy could do nothing to turn the tide. Homeopaths had been so spoiled by success that they expected history to deliver them whole. He wrote in his final report:

> He who sits comfortably in his easy chair in his smoking jacket enjoying a genuine Havana bought with silver earned by means of a successful homeopathic prescription, grunting a "Cui bono?" when called upon to do his share toward the perpetuation of the homeopathic doctrine, and he who vainly asserts that "Similia is a mighty truth and cannot die, no matter whether I get busy on its behalf or not!" letting it go at that, are likely to awaken some wintry morn to find themselves undeceived.[13]

In fact, that day had already come.

Meanwhile, mainstream medicine, with its organizing body, the AMA, and the *JAMA*, had a unique authority in relation to the sectarian medical schools. Having taken the sectarians into their mainstream, they now claimed a right to a say in such medical education, even though they were totally ignorant of its principles. Representing the new syncretist medicine, they sought to develop universal standards and criteria for practice. As long as there were two recognized competing medical traditions with two theories, the homeopaths were totally immune to interference from the allopaths, immune legally unless they were declared to be "quacks" by a recognized government body. When a significant proportion of homeopaths accepted general non-sectarian medicine—many of them innocently, thinking it was an inroad for homeopathy to be heard and tested in wider circles—the basis for a separate homeopathic training was forfeited.

In preparation for a grading of medical schools, the AMA developed a series of criteria for a good medical facility. These were absurdly biased against homeopathy, for they required nonpracticing research doctors (a contradiction in homeopathic terms), extensive laboratories (meaning pharmaceutical laboratories), and a balanced curriculum. The balanced curriculum was a web from which homeopathy could not extricate itself as long as it advanced its own methodology handed down by Hahnemann. It found itself isolated from both the American scientific tradition and professional etiquette.

In association with the Carnegie Foundation for the Advancement of Teaching, the AMA prepared a working paper on medical education in America and Canada. This study, issued in 1910 under the name of Abraham Flexner, the Carnegie representative, gave the AMA a basis for refusing licenses to the graduates of low-ranking institutions. Although ostensibly a temporary survey, the Flexner Report, rightly or wrongly, became the new basis on which medical education was organized. Modern medicine was recognized as the collection of the methods and theories that had proven effective *and* scientific. The sectarian schools were not immediately forced out of business, but they were permanently identified as "sectarian schools" rather than medical schools. Their attendance dropped, and during a period of time when orthodox medicine received substantial foundation funding and government support, they were left to their own fate. Over the years since, the gap has increased. Mainstream medicine has been lavishly funded; the sectarian schools have dwindled and all but disappeared. The Flexner Report said:

> ... now that allopathy has surrendered to modern medicine, is not homeopathy borne on the same current into the same harbor?
>
> For everything of proved value in homeopathy belongs of right to scientific medicine and is at this moment incorporate in it; nothing else has any footing at all, whether it be of allopathic or homeopathic lineage.[14]

Who could argue?

Seven homeopathic medical schools were left at the end of 1918; the Hahnemann Medical College of Philadelphia lasted until the 1920s, when it changed its orientation to allopathy. Homeopathic experiment, lacking a simple way to pose the problem of microdose, became as irrelevant and on the same basis as the alchemical experiment in transmutation of metals.

The decline of homeopathy changed the popular perception of disease categories. The emphasis fell away from chronic conditions, which were virtually untreatable anyway, onto severe disease and the demography of health, illness, and health care, where allopathy had the greatest success.

Chronic diseases were either passed on to specialists or declared undiagnosable and managed symptomatically. This process has reached its apex in modern medicine. The kinds of fees doctors have come to expect, after years of medical training, are not possible from the mere treatment of headaches and digestive difficulties, for example; many doctors have found it demeaning to be asked to solve such chronic cases, so they are dealt with in depth only by psychoanalysts, who come to link them with neuroses and other personality disorders prestigious and lucrative enough to "cure." We might exaggerate and say that in a certain sense only by becoming classified as mental illness can chronic diseases get respect. Even then, they are attacked often by psychotropics and held hostage by the fashions of the drug industry. If there were anything significant in Hahnemann's progression of chronic ailments or emotional-physical planes of disease, modern medicine is in no position to discover it.

From roughly 1910 until the late 1960s, few new homeopaths entered the ranks in the United States and Canada; as the last classes of homeopaths graduated from American medical schools in the 1920s and 1930s, only European-trained physicians were available. Homeopathy in North America had been consigned to the graveyard of medicine. The homeopathic community tended to accept their martyrdom; their mission was to keep the flame alive during these dark ages, to prevent it from being blown out altogether by the winds of materialism.

Ostensibly, during this time, the situation in Europe has been far more promising. Homeopathy continued as a viable medicine, with its hospitals and medical schools, throughout Western Europe, in the countries once part of the defunct British Empire, notably India, and in Chile and Argentina, where many German and Swiss immigrated. But it never achieved the dominance in these places that it did in America, and it is now a secondary medicine at best wherever it is practiced. Standards have deteriorated; far worse, there is controversy from country to country, and even from doctor to doctor, as to what constitutes acceptable homeopathic treatment.

Yet still, as Gorman writes, "... 32 percent of family physicians in France and 20 percent in Germany prescribe homeopathic medicines, while in Great Britain 42 percent sometimes refer patients to homeopaths. In France, where the best-selling flu remedy, Oscillococinum, is homeopathic, the national health-care system covers homeopathic prescriptions from traditional physicians."[15]

From a Hahnemannian perspective, homeopathy entered the 1970s as a dwindling collection of small national practices of mediocre and stagnant derivations and a handful of dying exiles in North America, perhaps individual prescribers of merit scattered throughout the world. Of course, the same landscape from a twentieth-century mainstream scientific perspective shows a successful universal medicine with some minor pockets of ignorant and superstitious resistance.

Developments of the last twenty years have altered the landscape significantly. There has been a resurgence of homeopathy in the United States; it is not yet significant in terms of absolute numbers, but it is unexpected in the context of the prior unchecked decline. It is also notable that in the last fifteen years, perhaps as many as a thousand new M.D.s have taken up homeopathic practice. In 1996 a survey of AMA primary-care physicians showed a surprising 49 percent interested in homeopathic training, 69 percent in a separate Maryland census. A homeopathic clinic began in Berkeley in the 1970s and continues to serve a growing number of clients. Homeopathic training programs, only four in 1990, were almost thirty in 1996. Additionally, 34 percent of all medical schools have training in alternative medicine in one form or another. As Mark Twain prophesized, "We may honestly feel grateful that homeopathy survived the attempts of the allopathists to destroy it."[16]

In April 1978 a major conference brought together homeopaths from around the United States, but mainly from west of the Rockies. George Vithoulkas flew from Greece to deliver fifteen hours of lectures to five hundred people at the California Academy of Sciences. At the end of this conference, the formation of an International Foundation for the Promotion of Homeopathy was announced, with the intention of raising standards of homeopathic practice throughout North America and the world. The founding directives included "strict scientific research on homeopathic potencies and their clinical application" and the establishment of full-time four-year homeopathic schools in Athens, Greece, and California.

The appearance in the San Francisco Bay Area of the most internationally renowned homeopath stimulated all the ambiguities that existed then in American homeopathy. The audience was made up of local Bay Area students and practitioners of homeopathy, older homeopaths from across the United States, and hundreds of doctors, lay prescribers, nurses, and patients, many of them practicing incognito. The underground movement was perhaps even stronger than was suspected. After Vithoulkas spoke at the University of California Hospital in San Francisco, he received a five-minute standing ovation from the medical personnel despite the fact that in his lecture everything that the medicine practiced in that building stood for he had demolished. At the Academy of Sciences, he was frequently interrupted with applause, sometimes for almost offhand descriptions of outdueling an allopath in a difficult case. At the high points of his talks, he was serenaded with "right on," as people stood and shook fists and gave V-signs.

For the older homeopaths there, it must have been a both disturbing and elating event, reversing their own strategy of fifty years. Never in their lifetime did they expect to see such an audience in praise of homeopathy. But it was not the audience they wanted. M.D.s with their hair in braids and in turbans and robes; country enthusiasts from Oregon, Idaho, Washington, Nevada, Utah, New Mexico, California, etc., dressed for the road or the farm, many bearded and long-haired. This was the social and political order Hahnemannian homeopathy had always stood against. In fact, the American Institute of Homeopathy long feared that an awakening of this sort would bring down the wrath of the AMA and Food and Drug Administration (FDA), which, to that point, was content to let homeopathy quietly die out. (Since 1938, when a homeopath in the United States Senate, Royal Copeland (D-NY), added the drugs in the *Homeopathic Pharmacopeia* to the list recognized by the FDA, microdoses have been legally protected. While they are deemed safe, of course the FDA has never tested their efficacy.) The audience at moments seemed inappropriate and threatening, especially when they appeared to cheer for the demise of specific allopathic patients.

136

Even as Vithoulkas was cheered, he warned the audience about their attitude. "Faddism," he said, "will give the momentary illusion of success, but it will lead even more swiftly to the end of this wonderful science than any amount of isolation."

A specially woven banner hung on the curtains behind the podium with the homeopathic logo (SIMILIA SIMILIBUS CURENTUR) stitched between two yellow calendulas. It was a medical lecture and ceremony both.

In the years since this conference, the old homeopathy has thrown off much of its cultlike history and esoteric reputation and reclothed itself in computerized offices with modern reference texts and well-trained personnel. The second coming of homeopathy has learned to boogie in the streets with other New Age businesses and therapies. A combination of professionalism, training programs in naturopathic and other colleges and schools, M.D. costuming and paraphernalia, and feel-good marketing has given homeopathy a totally new image. In many circles within our ecological and holistic ramage of subcultures, the cylindrical vial labeled "Aconite" or "Causticum" has become as recognizable a trademark as Kellogg's Corn Flakes once was—the medicine of choice. Homeopathy has even developed a chic Hollywood/*Rolling Stone* popularity, a far cry not only from Hahnemann's Paris clinic but also Vithoulkas' proud apocalypticism. Homeopathic pharmacies are now recommended in socially conscious, post-yuppie portfolios.

Meanwhile, research toward legitimacy has continued:

> Recently, the *British Medical Journal* published an eight-page review of 25 years of clinical research on homeopathy. This meta-analysis was completed by three Dutch epidemiologists who were commissioned by their government as the result of an earlier study which indicated that 45 percent of Dutch physicians consider homeopathic medicines to be effective. It uncovered a total of 107 controlled clinical trials, 81 of which showed the efficacy of homeopathic medicines. The researchers carefully evaluated each of these experiments and determined that 22 studies were of a particularly high quality in terms of their research design and the number of subjects used. Fifteen of these 22 studies showed

the efficacy of the homeopathic medicines. These trials indicated the range of successes that homeopaths commonly observe, including the effective treatment of arthritis, migraine headaches, allergies and hay fever, influenza, respiratory infections, postoperative infections, injuries, and childbirth.

The researchers concluded that "the amount of positive evidence even among the best studies came as a surprise to us.... The evidence presented in this review would probably be sufficient for establishing homeopathy as a regular treatment for certain conditions."

In a well-controlled, double-blind study of patients with hay fever which was published in the *Lancet*, Reilly et al. showed that the 30c of a mixture of 12 common pollens in the Glasgow area was very successful in reducing symptoms of hay fever.[17]

In 1980, the *British Journal of Clinical Pharmacology* published a double-blind study of patients with rheumatoid arthritis.[18] The study showed that 82 percent of those who had been given an individually chosen homeopathic medicine experienced some relief of symptoms, while only 21 percent of those who had been given a placebo experienced a similar degree of improvement.

In addition to these and numerous clinical trials, there are also dozens of laboratory experiments.[19] A study, published in *Human Toxicology*, replicated earlier work and showed that homeopathic doses of arsenic helped rats excrete through their urine and feces the crude doses they earlier had been given.[20] This study also used radioactive tracers to evaluate efficacy of the microdose. Ultimately, the 7c and 14x were found to have the greatest benefit. The implications of this work are quite significant when one considers the environmental exposures that humans and animals commonly experience today.

Those skeptics who many years ago said that homeopathy had no research basis were obviously unfamiliar with a double-blind study in 1944 funded by the British government which evaluated the homeopathic treatment of mustard gas burns.[21] This research showed that *Rhus Tox 30c*, *Mustard Gas 30c*, and *Kali Bichromicum 330c* each provided benefit when compared with placebo treatment.

Other early well-controlled studies include some 1942 research by the Scottish physician W. E. Boyd and his work using enzyme diastase in starch hydrolysis.[22] He showed that hydrolysis was accelerated using the enzyme inhibitor mercuric chloride at 61x, while hydrolysis was inhibited at lower potencies. This work was done so meticulously that it was strongly praised by an associate dean of an American medical school.

Singh and Gupta demonstrated antiviral action in eight of ten homeopathic medicines tested on chicken embryo virus.[23] Between 50–100 percent inhibition was common for these drugs. A similar test of four medicines on Similike Forest Virus (a virus that causes paralysis in mice) showed that none had any observable effect as compared with the control.

Several studies have shown that homeopathic medicines can control fungal and viral diseases in plants.[24] [(25)]

(See also the discussion of I_E crystals on pages 80–81.)

In 1997 almost two thousand conventionally trained M.D.s practiced homeopathy in the United States; another three to five thousand health professionals, including dentists and nurses, are also primarily homeopathic in their drug use. Add to these some five thousand chiropractors who include homeopathic remedy selection in their practices and an untold number of lay practitioners and consumers who individualize medicines from books and kits with only the most informal or indirect training.[26]

Every domain within the field has grown in kind—courses, publications, self-help kits, pharmacies, even software for both IBM and Macintosh systems for the professional homeopath, and an IBM-compatible system for the consumer to self-treat a range of common ailments from the voluminous homeopathic materia medica.[26]

During the last fifteen years, sales of homeopathic medicines have increased by 25 percent a year in the United States.[26]

Could this all be placebo and delusion? It is hard to believe that so many people could be involved in a practice that did not result in some sort of concrete health improvement.

Of course, the greening of homeopathy has disseminated within a larger holistic-health movement. Technological medicine has achieved its late twentieth-century destiny through overwhelming HMOs and strict patient counts. As one M.D. put it, "We are in a new dark age of medicine." People are frightened and alienated by a machinery that dwarfs and trivializes their humanity and takes the power of their own health out of their hands. They seek simple and personal alternatives.

The early history of naturopathic medicine in America is now repeating itself. Whereas a century and a half ago homeopathy was practiced in the context of native herbal medicines, now it has been encompassed in an amalgam of therapies that is collectively far vaster and more diverse. The new homeopathy is first and foremost an integral part of a syncretized system of native American herbal, Third World herbal, and Eurasian scientific pharmacies that provides a medicine chest of substances tested empirically in a variety of climates and for periods ranging from decades to millennia, all integrated into a single neo-alchemical, osteopathic discourse of diagnosis and treatment. Homeopathic medicines are commercially indistinguishable from Chinese herbal blends, Bach flower remedies (which are also spiritualized), and various ultra-modern vitamin compounds that would do Johnson & Johnson proud.

Many people only know of homeopathy through the advertised, occasionally overnamed formulas that blend many microdoses into one remedy. These formulas are obviously not individualized according to a unique pattern of symptoms. They are sold for anyone's "PMS," headaches, flu, back pain, allergies, digestive problems, etc., much as allopathic drugs are. Modern homeopaths generally argue that either a synergy or catchall effect occurs when, for instance, the ingredients for treating five different allergies are combined. In any case, this may be the only way the general public ever gets to try out homeopathic remedies. The formulas are clearly marketing tools in an era in which packaging threatens to supersede product. However, to say that they oversimplify homeopathic diagnosis and treatment overlooks the dilemma that until we know how homeopathic remedies work, we cannot limit the range of their preparation and application. Formulas *seem* to work. As long as a variety of alternative pharmacies and energy medicines are made available, people are going to test the boundaries of an unknown system embracing psychic as well as physical and even cultural variables. The era of worshipping technological synthesis as the "miracle drug" factory is over. The era of seeking a new paradigm among microdoses, meridians, chakras, and natural sources of immunity is now underway.

As general holistic therapeutics, homeopathy is also practiced in the company of cranial osteopathy, Feldenkrais bodywork, rebirthing, acupuncture, polarity, *chi gung,* macrobiotic and other highly conscious diets, as well as at consumer-oriented clinics that have some strong allopathic persuasions. Homeopathy is part of a new shamanic, somatic, psychoanalytic, energy-based, self-reflective, gender-conscious, and ethnically diverse "planet medicine." Within that nexus, it has its own science-fiction story to tell. Medicine aside, the cultural situation is provocative enough that *The New York Times Magazine* was receptive to James Gorman's article. In keeping with his educated but cynical audience, Gorman opens with a description of a revival that must have seemed to some readers like a rebirth of witchcraft on the New York Stock Exchange. While everyone in his milieu, including himself, was asleep, homeopathy "jus' grew." Suddenly Gorman finds that:

> ... almost everyone I knew either had used a homeopathic remedy or knew someone who did. Drugstores that a few years ago were carrying only mainstream products like Nyquil and Sudafed were displaying homeopathic lines in their windows. And not in amber bottles, but in small, colorful cardboard containers with the pills comfortably ensconced in blister packs. There was Quietude—"the homeopathic insomnia remedy" in a white box with blue and pink pastel borders. And Alpha CF, for colds and flu, in an icy-blue package with a snowflake design.
>
> I was not the only one to notice that homeopathy was in vogue and visually more attractive than ever. A newspaper article about an up-and-coming bicoastal style monger named Andre Balazs noted that a feature planned for the ultra-chic Manhattan hotel he's building is a homeopathic pharmacy. If it does well, Balazs envisions a chain.
>
> This would obviously please the homeopathic pharmaceutical companies, which are already undergoing a renaissance. Old companies are reviving, and new companies are getting into the field, which in the late 1970s and early 1980s made a miraculous recovery from near death. According to the Food and Drug Administration, sales of some homeopathic drug companies

increased 1,000 percent. Growth has continued apace ever since, with the American market for homeopathic drugs now estimated at [$150] million.

Europe's [three] biggest homeopathic pharmaceutical companies have moved into the United States, each acquiring a struggling old American firm. Boiron L.H.F., of France, a publicly held company, bought Borneman & Sons of Philadelphia in 1983. In 1987 the privately owned Dr. Willmar Schwabe GmbH & Company, of Germany, purchased Boericke & Tafel, another Philadelphia company, founded in 1825, and in 1990 moved it into a new, state-of-the-art production facility in Santa Rosa, California. Both companies report that gross sales have increased by more than 20 percent a year, a claim matched by Standard Homeopathic Company, an old-line California firm. [Dolisos, France's second-largest company, recently opened an American office.]

New to the homeopathic market is Nature's Way Products Inc., a manufacturer of food supplements, which describes itself as "America's Natural Health Care Company." The full-page magazine advertisements trumpeting its new line of homeopathic medicines assure consumers that they "work a lot like vaccines" and are easy to use. "If my back hurts, I get the remedy labeled for injury and backache, and there's one for arthritis, PMS, colds or whatever. It's simple." So simple, in fact, that there is a remedy labeled simply "allergy."

Imagine—medicines that have no side effects, so safe that a child could swallow an entire bottle of pills, yet able to cure picky ailments like fatigue, insomnia and [allergies] that have baffled modern medicine. How could such medicines be produced? What went into them?...

Boericke & Tafel's brand-new headquarters seemed the best place to look on the new face of homeopathy, so I flew to San Francisco and then drove north to Santa Rosa. The plant was spanking clean, just the way you want a pharmaceutical plant to be. In the laboratory-like production rooms, everyone (including me) wore white coats, surgical masks and gloves and disposable caps.... The workers also put on special white shoes, which they wore only while in these areas. Visitors and all other personnel were given covers for theirs. (The last time I had seen people dressed this way was at my son's birth.) In one area a tablet-making machine was busy making tablets. In another, the tincture storage room, there were scores of amber bottles on stainless-steel racks, all very pharmaceutical. But there was no amoxycillin or Prozac, no Xanax or AZT. Instead there were tinctures of Rhus radicans (poison ivy), Berberis vulgaris (barberry) and Calcarea silicata (silicate of lime). In another area, Calendula officinalis (marigold) was macerating in what seemed to be large stainless-steel stockpots.

Next we entered the "single remedy room," where medicines were actually being produced. First the technician weighed out a gram's worth of drops from one bottle of Natrum muriaticum 25X. Otherwise known as sodium chloride or table salt, the Natrum muriaticum had been diluted 25 times at a ratio of 1 to 10, leaving 1 part salt to 10 to the 25th power parts of alcohol and water (10 followed by 25 zeros, a number so high that the name used to describe it is a "googol"). After each dilution the solution was shaken 10 times by hand and banged against a rubber pad, a process known in homeopathy as "succussion." In homeopathy this process of diluting, shaking and banging is known as "potentizing." In homeopathic speak the solution was at 25X potency.

To this already ethereal solution the technician added more liquid to dilute it 1 to 10 once again. She then succussed the solution by shaking it 10 times by hand (up and down) and banging it against a rubber pad on each down stroke. The solution was now Natrum muriaticum 26X. She repeated the same procedure again to produce a 27X solution. The final steps (done later) would be to repeat the dilution and succussion process three more times to achieve Natrum muriaticum 30X. Then drops of this solution of 1 part salt to 10 to the 30th power parts liquid would be added to sugar tablets, resulting in a product reputedly useful for allergy, anemia, cardiovascular problems and grieving states.

As I watched this process I heard within me the whimper of offended reason. By all known laws of physics and chemistry, the initial preparation had been diluted so many times that it was highly unlikely that a measurable trace of salt remained, not a molecule. And this was before the five succeeding dilutions, and the final dosing of the sugar pellets. What was being created, it seemed, was not a drug, but the idea of a drug, what an artist friend of mine calls "conceptual medicine." I thought, Welcome to homeopathy.[27]

It is sufficient for us to note that medicine is presently at a cross-roads in the United States. The homeopathic revival is part of a cultural rebellion against the authoritarianism and sterility of the "M.D." cult of the last generation. A cohesive, self-consistent system has not yet emerged. Different levels and types of homeopathy are inevitable as long as basic contradictions within the system and the practice are unresolved. What is clear is that, from the beginning, homeopathy has been a process working toward something millennial and important. That process will press on through the different forms and versions until that something is manifested. The mere hope of an inexpensive and effective cure, for whatever reason, should keep us satisfied till then.

Appendix 1

A Case History

The paradox of homeopathy as well as the opportunity it poses is depicted by a case that developed in my own family fifteen years ago. My wife, Lindy, and I went through a baffling three-year-long ailment with our daughter Miranda, then nine years old.

Miranda's ailment surfaced in September of 1983 with a boil (sty) on her left eye after a cold. It took two weeks of soaking to break it open; a fairly typical "pink eye" infection followed, spreading to both eyes. When the infection persisted for another week, we took her to our GP, a doctor sympathetic to homeopathy and other alternative treatments and, in fact, an editor of holistic-health books. He prescribed an antibiotic (Erythromyocin), after which the "pink eye" improved. However, her eyes never really felt right; they itched and were red in the mornings. She had times, especially at school, when she wanted only to close them, so that we periodically had to fetch her home. Since it was a new and difficult school for which she wasn't fully prepared, we and the GP gave some consideration to a psychological influence. (She also has large, light blue eyes that have always attracted attention.)

One Sunday morning in February Miranda had shooting pains in both eyes. They grew so uncomfortable that eventually she rolled on the floor. We met a substitute for our GP at his office. He could find no visible sign of infection but, in testing her vision, found that it had deteriorated significantly since September. He sent us

145

to the only ophthalmologist who would see her at once. We ended up at a crowded clinic filled with young children and elderly people. After a several-hour wait, the doctor examined her with eye charts and slit lamps. Based on her poor vision at the time, he was mainly interested in prescribing glasses. He did see signs of an infection, but he downplayed it as secondary to her vision and prescribed a stronger antibiotic with a steroid. He assured us the infection would go away in two weeks.

Although Miranda had no further acute attacks in those two weeks, her eyes still bothered her. She described it mainly as a sensation of something being stuck in them. She did not want to open them in bright light, and often when we were outdoors, she would pretend to be blind and ask to be led—a game that amused her and frightened us.

We kept our two-week appointment, at which the ophthalmologist declared the infection cured; he then of course wanted to proceed with glasses. We decided to wait. Meanwhile, the physician mother of one of Miranda's friends told us that we should be concerned about systemic diseases. We called a relative who is a gynecologist in San Francisco. He recommended an ophthalmologist from New York who, he said, was the best children's eye doctor in the Bay Area; he even set up the first appointment for us within a week.

This prominent physician seemed both compassionate and knowledgeable. He said almost immediately, "This is a very uncomfortable little girl and for good reason." After a thorough examination, he told us that the original ophthalmologist didn't know what he was talking about; Miranda had an extensive infection that had left disease products in her eyes and mottled the corneas. He prescribed regular cleansing of the vicinity around the eyes with a Q-tip and shampoo (the brand name No Tears, which Miranda came to call More Tears), and a stronger antibiotic with cortisone.

To this point we had made no attempt to find an alternative physician. The disease was in a risky area, had begun as a "simple" infection, and had generated its own trail of doctors. We were not naive about deeper causes, but much of life is spent not dealing with the real source of things. Miranda was already in a situation of having trouble keeping up in school, and there seemed little room in which to experiment, especially with her eyes. This is typical of the circumstance in which most health care is sought and dispensed—like heading into the nearest fast-food outlet when you're hungry because there is only an hour before you're due back at work. It's why most people postpone self-inquiry and change, often forever. One is inattentive until their dilemma is so serious they are jolted to responsiveness.

When systemic illness became a possibility, my first hope for a resolution was homeopathy. However, when the heralded ophthalmologist dismissed the possibility of more serious disease—and later confirmed his dismissal by lab tests—I returned to my distraction, neglecting homeopathic axioms about disease layers. The continuation of an antibiotic, now amplified by cortisone, was certainly unwelcome by any holistic standards, but we resolved to use it for as brief a time as possible. The credentials of our doctor led us to believe that the disease would soon be resolved, at least on the symptomatic level.

Miranda began a daily regimen of cleaning and applying the antibiotic. Her improvement—if any—was minor, but at least she did not have any recurrences of acute and painful attacks. During the summer she complained about her eyes sweating and the effect on them of traffic fumes and even perfume which, she said, caused them to "go crazy." She demonstrated with frenzied jigs. She was still hypersensitive to light and avoided the sun. We finally made another appointment in August. The ophthalmologist reexamined her thoroughly and said, despite her complaints, that he saw no further sign of infection. It was only a matter of time, he felt, before all effects of the disease disappeared. He told her to continue scrubbing scrupulously.

During the first weeks of school Miranda's problems got considerably worse. She ended up sitting by the side with her eyes closed on several occasions, and either Lindy or I were summoned to rescue her.

We insisted on another ophthalmological appointment, which we took Miranda to directly from school one day. The once-charming venerable physician was definitely frayed; he accused us of not following through on his treatments because we believed in alternative medicines and insisted that her relapse was our fault (he did finally agree that the infection was still raging). He referred us immediately to a San Francisco clinic specializing in infectious diseases of the eye.

Miranda's examination and culture there cost $200, and we were told that she had an allergological reaction to an underlying infection. There was no cure for the complex, but it could be treated hygienically. This meant continuing the shampoo treatments, but extending them to the nostrils and the sides of the nose. The doctor at the clinic emphasized that all of our previous treatments had been either wrong or incomplete. The original Erythromyocin was the only antibiotic to which the bacteria were susceptible, and the antibiotics prescribed by both ophthalmologists were incorrect and, in the case of the cortisone, contraindicated and potentially blindness-causing! The cleaning would work only if she got all the infected zones, which meant her entire face and scalp. Otherwise bacteria would simply spread again from the ignored pockets.

Still stung by the earlier doctor's accusations, we implemented that treatment rigorously for three and a half months into December. The condition improved enough that Miranda was able to stay at school and keep her eyes open, but she was unable to participate in outdoor sports in direct light (thus sat on the side), and still had very red eyes in the morning and a great deal of difficulty stretching them open. At this point we assumed that allopathy could make no further headway, and we allowed a lay homeopath to take her case. He prescribed *Pulsatilla* on a constitutional basis. He also asked us to discontinue the topical antibiotic for at least ten days, advising us that she might experience an immediate aggravation. She developed a heavy cold, but her eyes neither improved nor got worse.

Later in the month we were in northern rural California and visited a macrobiotic naturopath we already knew. He suggested eliminating all dairy products, plus carrying out a mild saltwater bathing of the eyes twice daily, including snorting through her nostrils. He felt Miranda's sodium balance was off, and he specifically prescribed a complete mineral salt to improve that balance as well as to make up for what he called other trace-element deficiencies. He said that homeopathy, for using just one substance at a time, could never fulfill the range of needs in her system. It was a misunder-standing of homeopathy, but even complementarily vitalistic sys-tems sometimes can be incompatible.

After two weeks Miranda's eyes were itchy and red *and* it was time for her to return to school; we were at a new impasse. We did not want to antidote the homeopathic treatment, but we needed something to control the discomfort, so we returned to the Ery-thromyocin while continuing the bathing and restrictive diet. A few days later the right eye was clear, but the left eye was swollen almost shut. We called the clinic and they said there was nothing we could do but persist in the treatment. We called the prior ophthal-mologist, and he said that the swelling was an infection in the gland and to continue soaking it. At this point we were back where we had begun, though with a much worse situation.

I phoned an out-of-town homeopath and described Miranda's history and condition in detail. With much reservation about remote prescribing he mailed us *Tuberculinum 30* and included a letter in which he described her condition as a deep-seated inherited psoric miasm and warned that use of the remedy with the antibiotic would eventually cause mutual aggravation. Within days after we gave the remedy, the sty went down, but a second sty formed on the upper eyelid and swelled to the size of a marble. We continued to soak it, but there was no improvement and she could not go to school.

We returned to our GP. He felt that whatever else was true that he had to prescribe an oral antibiotic to deal with the immediate infection. She took Tetracycline, and the sty eventually broke, although two months later it was still present in reduced form. During those months she continued the hygienic treatment and occasionally used topical Erythromyocin. (The out-of-town home-opath later attributed the failure of the remedy to the fact that she mistakenly took it twice—in his mind a very dangerous action. ("It's lucky," he said, "it was her eye and not her heart.")

In early March the situation escalated. Miranda bumped into her brother Robin in the hall and struck her eye. She screamed for almost ten minutes and said she wanted to die. I called my gyne-cologist cousin and reviewed the alternatives. The next morning he rang me back, having gotten us an appointment with a research ophthalmologist who did not ordinarily see patients but nonetheless would meet us in his laboratory that afternoon.

He was a distinguished-looking gentleman, near retirement, more gentle with Miranda than any of the practicing physicians had been. With a graduate student, he ran her through the battery of slit lamps, dyes, and cultures and then heard out our whole history, which included naturopathy and homeopathy. He said he knew her condition and could understand our series of blind circles. The disease was essentially—as the clinic had explained—a special reaction to ordinary bacteria. But he was more precise: It wasn't an infection of the eye in the usual sense and certainly should not have been treated as conjunctivitis; it was possibly the result of a preadolescent acne so slight as to be almost imperceptible except for an oiliness and slight scaling around the nose. The bacterial by-products of the skin got into the eyelids, lashes, and onto the cornea itself, causing the scarring. Through his magnifying lenses I could see the stained surface of Miranda's cornea with pits and streamers of irritation. "Deep-seated psoric miasm indeed," he mused. "The language is not contemporary, but the diagnosis is essentially correct. I wouldn't say anything when my student was here because he'd have my head. Graduate students are so narrow these days. But she has inherited a complex to which she is unable to generate a normal immune response."

We went back to the regimen of washing and using a topical ointment. Miranda visited the laboratory every other week; her vision was tested, the surface of her eyes mapped, her face photographed, and a culture taken each time. "I'm the star," she remarked after one session. Another time she added, "There's no cure. I'm going to be like this forever. He'll have a photo album of my whole life."

Soon there was gradual if not overwhelming improvement in the scarring at the surface of the cornea and her discomfort. The photophobia and irritation remained. Her vision stabilized at the level to which it had initially declined, serious enough for glasses if it remained but not debilitating in most circumstances.

Three months into this treatment she suddenly developed *acne rosaceae*. We were now truly trapped between systems of medicine. A homeopath friend said that we had to let the acne run its course because it was the externalization of the disease into less vital organs. The research ophthalmologist said, "Hogwash! The acne is the source of the infection, and it is now rampant. Unless we treat this immediately with an internal antibiotic her sight will be threatened."

We agreed to let her take Tetracycline. For his part the ophthalmologist promised the smallest possible amount—"an almost homeopathic dose," he joked. At the same time we went to see the one homeopath in our area who would work with patients using allopathic drugs. On the day Miranda started the Tetracycline, he took the entire case and prescribed a homeopathic remedy—*Mercurius.* It was a very low potency—6C—but he had her take it three times daily. He also prescribed homeopathically prepared microdoses of Tetracycline, to diminish negative side effects from the drug. I asked him the obvious questions: wasn't the skin ailment a movement outward of the disease? Won't the antibiotic and potency aggravate each other? Isn't giving repeated doses dangerous? He said: "I'm not an ideologue."

He was interested in treating Miranda as she was. Her sight was threatened, so she should be taking an antibiotic. "A good homeopathic treatment isn't bound to rules," he added. "I'm involved only in restoring her actual vital force. I've never had any problems with antibiotics or multiple doses, and I consider such homeopathy pure superstition."

During a month of travel on the East Coast, Miranda took all three remedies—a foul-tasting fungus and two sugar pills containing only spiritualized essence—and continued to scrub. She experienced the most dramatic improvement yet. Her skin cleared completely, she was able to be outside in bright sunlight for the first time in months, and when we returned, her bacteria level was down and her cornea less aggravated. The ophthalmologist thought the Tetracycline did it, but admitted he didn't know how. "I gave it to her in subtherapeutic doses, and she missed a number of days at that. It's really a black box. Maybe homeopathic mercury is the answer, but I won't write that down anywhere. Who cares, as long as she's better?"

When I remarked that it was too bad we couldn't tell what had cured her, he said with a smile, "Oh, Son of Man, thou canst not know."

That spring he expressed some disappointment that, despite other improvement, the cornea was still pitted and Miranda's vision hadn't improved. Seemingly independently, she had developed plantar's warts, and they had spread along her feet and become quite painful. With reduction of sensitivity in her eyes, she had begun ballet, and the warts made movement difficult. Lindy wanted to have a dermatologist treat them, as was done in her childhood; I felt that they were somehow connected to the antibiotic and the eyes and I wanted the homeopath to see her.

We compromised. Miranda went first to a dermatologist, who said that the warts were deep-seated and would be difficult to remove without surgery. The next day she went to the homeopath. In taking her case anew he repetorized a remedy that covered both scarring of the cornea and plantar's warts (*Silica*), and he prescribed it. He then observed that *Mercurius* had been selected primarily for photophobia, which it seemed to have already handled.

Within twenty-four hours the plantar's warts had turned black and begun to fall off; a week later the ophthalmologist found her cornea remarkably cleared, and on the eye chart she shot right through the 20/20 line and kept on going until he said, with a smile, it was good enough.

The actual course of this disease and its treatments is a map of something unknown. Since we have no information about how either subtherapeutic Tetracycline or microdoses of *Mercurius* and *Silica* work in tissue, or how Miranda's own metabolism and individuating psyche affected all this, we can resolve nothing vis-à-vis competing systems, nor did we have any guarantee the cure would be sustained.

In fact, the ailment came back ten years later at age twenty-one and is proving difficult to treat two years hence. *Silica* and *Mercurius* had no effect this time. Craniosacral therapy, notably adjustments freeing the movement of the sphenoid bone behind the eyes, was successful in relieving an associated headache and a feeling of tightness in the skull. Acupuncture and Chinese herbs have also seemed to improve mental and circulatory aspects while, if anything, exacerbating the immune response in the eyes.

All medicine works in league with a mystery. Homeopathy accentuates that mystery by reducing the concrete to the nonmaterial and the symptom to its molecular origin.

But, each time, we find ourselves at a new level. Each time we must "take the case" again and treat what is expressing itself now. There is no end to emergence, evolution, and unfolding.

Can we someday provide the same "canst not know" cure for the ancient ecosystems that alone ensure the continuity of cell life on the Earth?

Can we restore the mystery of the unconscious, the microdose, the Similar, to the ponds, meadows, oceans, jungles, and skies of a world overwhelmed with the toxic by-products of its sheer materiality, its externalization (and assembly-line replication) of a pathology at the heart of our species (from which all creatures, plant and animal, now flee)?

It is no longer just the problem of worried citizens seeking capable doctors themselves awash among contradicting paradigms and impossible futures. It is the dilemma of our whole civilization.

Appendix 2

A Comparison of
Homeopathy to Other Modalities

In summary, **homeopathy** resembles a number of other medicinal practices but is strikingly distinct from all of them in major ways.

Homeopathy resembles **herbal medicine** in that it is primarily botanical and ethnopharmaceutical. It differs from herbal medicine insofar as it uses microdoses (spiritualized or quantal doses) in place of molecularly active substances.

Homeopathy resembles **Ayurvedic (East Indian) pharmacy** in that it employs animal, vegetable, and mineral substances medicinally according to constitutional interpretations and in that it prescribes remedies according to empirically derived psychosomatic characterologies. It differs from Ayurveda in its emphasis on minute doses and algebraic preparations but also in its development of a repertory of symptoms and types according to a Western method of taxonomy and in its relatively small sample of patients for repertorizing (a few centuries rather than a few millennia).

Homeopathy resembles **Chinese acupuncture and moxibustion** (and to some degree, Chinese herbs) in its emphasis on a dynamic, vitalized field state, transcending ordinary laws of matter; the transmission of a cure in the form of energy; and in its constitutional theory. Homeopathy differs from Chinese medicine in its emphasis on infinite character permutations rather than elemental (ying/yang) cycles; its generally impalpable, clinical application (no doctor-patient physical contact); and its algebraic pharmacy.

Homeopathy resembles **osteopathy** (including **chiropractic** and **craniosacral therapy**) in its seeming morphogenetic activation of visceral and emotional changes along a spreading hierarchy of fractal tissue levels from a simple, singular point of contact. It differs from all mechanical medicines in its use of a pill rather than palpation or manipulation to activate its point of contact, its character types in place of visceral configurations, and its emphasis on instantaneous transmission rather than neuromuscular, hydrostatic, or cellular transmission.

Homeopathy resembles **allopathy** (standard medicine) in its shared history going back to the Arabs, Greeks, and Romans, including a lineage of medical schools that taught both allopathy and homeopathy until recently; its use of statistical and scientific methods; its clinical doctor-patient grids; and its commitment to a biophysical rationale. It differs from allopathy in its priority of empiricism over rationalism, its spiritualized pharmacy, its distinction between disease core and layers of symptoms at different states of materiality, its treatment by Similars rather than antidotes, its theosophical metaphysics, and its grand theory of disease and civilization.

Homeopathy resembles **psychiatry** in its recognition of the psychosomatic basis and emotional components of all disease and the importance of treating from the psychological roots outward to physical embodiments. It also resembles psychiatry in its transference-like elicitation of symptoms. It differs from psychiatry in its total lack of interest in destructuring neurosis or finding an affective basis for behavior. Homeopathy uses psychological elements in its diagnosis but not in the mechanics of its treatment. Like Chinese medicine, Ayurveda, shamanism, osteopathy, and other holistic medicines, it presumes that body, mind, and spirit come together in instantaneous recognition and transmission at the moment of the correct treatment.

Homeopathy resembles **shamanism** in its magical relationship between remedy and healer, substance (or symbol) and patient, and healer and patient (especially when a medicine is transmitted psychically). Homeopathic succussion also suggests the dynamizing features of chanting, drumming, and evocative masks. But homeopathy is a modernized, utterly clinical version of shamanic principles. It buries its totems, spirits, were-bears, and were-ravens in the place the civilized world prefers them—in sanitized offices where they are quantized, commoditized, and neutrally dispensed.

Homeopathy resembles **alchemy** in its apparent transmutation of substance; it differs from alchemy in that it uses a decimal-based, microcosmic, nonelemental, simplified method of transmutation. It also differs insofar as it is based on a miasmatic theory of civilization and disease rather than on a Gnostic view of the evolution of spirit through minerals. Homeopathy is more botanical than mineral because it includes but does not sanctify or mythologize the alchemical hierarchies of mineral spirits. Homeopathy represents a transmutation and rebirth of alchemy after the first demythologizing wave of the scientific revolution. It *is* alchemy, but in the context of zero-based mathematics and chemistry.

Homeopathy also shares some aspects of the energizing of matter, the concentration of potency in microdoses, and the fusion of emotions and dynamized substance with many other alternative modalities, including **aromatherapy, Bach flower remedies, healing by color, sound therapy, Polarity**, and **orgone therapy**.

Homeopathic Resources

HOMEOPATHIC ORGANIZATIONS

National Center for Homeopathy
  801 N. Fairfax #306
  Alexandria, VA 22314   (703) 548-7790
  http://www.homeopathic.org

International Foundation for Homeopathy
  P.O. Box 7
  Edmonds, WA 98020   (425) 776-4147

Foundation for Homeopathic Education and Research
  2124 Kittredge St.
  Berkeley, CA 94704   (510) 649-8930

American Institute of Homeopathy
  925 E. 17th Ave.
  Denver, CO 80220   (303) 321-4105

Homeopathic Academy of Naturopathic Physicians
  14653 S. Graves Road
  Mulino, OR 97042

American Homeopathic Pharmacists Association
  P.O. Box 80178
  Valley Forge, PA 19484   (610) 735-5124

SOURCES OF HOMEOPATHIC MEDICINES

The following companies either manufacture homeopathic medicines or provide a mail-order service for them. Homeopathic medicines are also commonly available at health food stores and pharmacies, though the following list of companies provides a more extensive assortment of homeopathic remedies.

Biological Homeopathic Industries
    11600 Cochiti S.E.
    Albuquerque, NM 87123   (505) 293-3843

Boericke and Tafel
    2381 Circadian Way
    Santa Rosa, CA 95407 (707) 571-8202

Boiron-Bornemann, Inc.
    6 Campus Blvd., Building A
    Newtown Square, PA 19073   (610) 325-7464
    also: 98c W. Cochran
    Simi Valley, CA 93065   (805) 582-9091

Dolisos
    3014 Rigel Road
    Las Vegas, NV 89102   (702) 871-7153

Homeopathic Educational Services
    2124 Kittredge St.
    Berkeley, CA 94704   (510) 649-0294
    http://www.homeopathic.com

Luyties Pharmacal
    4200 Laclede Ave.
    St. Louis, MO 63108   (314) 533-9600

Standard Homeopathic Company
    204–210 W. 131st St.
    Los Angeles, CA 90061   (310) 321-4284

BOOKS ON HOMEOPATHY

Introductory Books and Family Guidebooks

Cummings, Stephen, and Dana Ullman. *Everybody's Guide to Homeopathic Medicines*. New York: Tarcher/Putnam, 1997.

Kruzel, Thomas. *Homeopathic Emergency Guide*. Berkeley: North Atlantic, 1992.

Lockie, Andrew. *The Family Guide to Homeopathy*. New York: Fireside, 1993.

Ullman, Dana. *The Consumer's Guide to Homeopathy*. New York: Jeremy P. Tarcher/Putnam 1996.

Ullman, Dana. *Discovering Homeopathy*. Berkeley: North Atlantic, 1991.

Ullman, Robert, and Judyth Reichenberg-Ullman. *The Quick and Easy Guide to Homeopathic Self-Care*. Rocklin, CA: Prima, 1996.

Specialized Self-Care Books

Bailey, Philip. *Homeopathic Psychology: Personality Profiles of the Major Homeopathic Remedies*. Berkeley: North Atlantic, 1995.

Castro, Miranda. *The Homeopathic Guide to Stress*. New York: St. Martin's, 1995.

Chappel, Peter. *Emotional Healing with Homeopathy*. Rockport, MA: Element, 1994.

Herscu, Paul. *The Homeopathic Treatment of Children: Pediatric Constitutional Types*. Berkeley: North Atlantic, 1991.

Hershoff, Asa. *Homeopathy for Musculoskeletal Healing*. Berkeley: North Atlantic, 1996.

Lockie, Andrew, and Nicola Geddes. *The Women's Guide to Homeopathy*. New York: St. Martin's, 1994.

Moskowitz, Richard. *Homeopathic Medicine for Pregnancy and Childbirth*. Berkeley: North Atlantic, 1992.

Souter, Keith. *Homoeopathy for the Third Age*. Saffron, Walden, England: C.W. Daniel, 1993.

Subotnick, Steven. *Sports and Exercise Injuries: Conventional, Homeopathic, and Alternative Treatments*. Berkeley: North Atlantic, 1991.

Ullman, Dana. *Homeopathic Medicine for Children and Infants.*
New York: Jeremy P. Tarcher/Putnam, 1992.

Ullman, Robert, and Judyth Reichenberg-Ullman. *Ritalin-Free Kids*, Rocklin, CA: Prima, 1994.
(See also Notes, page 166.)

Science and Research

Paolo Bellavite and Andrea Signorini, *Homeopathy: A Frontier in Medical Science*, Berkeley: North Atlantic, 1995.

See also *The Consumer's Guide to Homeopathy* by Dana Ullman, M.P.H. New York: Jeremy P. Tarcher/Putnam, 1995.

History of Homeopathy

Coulter, Harris L. *Divided Legacy: A History of the Schism in Medical Thought* (4 volumes). Berkeley: North Atlantic, 1975, 1977, 1981, 1994. Of special interest to people interested in the history of homeopathy is volume III: *Divided Legacy: The Conflict Between Homoeopathy and the American Medical Association.*

Notes

Chapter One

1. James Gorman, "Take a Little Deadly Nightshade and You'll Feel Better," *The New York Times Magazine* (August 30, 1992): 26.
2. Dana Ullman, "Homeopathic Medicine: A Modern View," *Whole Earth Review*, Fall, 1993. Material quoted from expanded prepublication version.

Chapter Two

1. *Hippocrates*, translated by W. H. S. Jones; quoted in Harris L. Coulter, *Divided Legacy, A History of the Schism in Medical Thought, Volume I: The Patterns Emerge: Hippocrates to Paracelsus* (Washington, D.C.: Wehawken Book Company, 1975): 77.
2. Coulter, *Divided Legacy I*, 89.
3. Coulter, *Divided Legacy I*, 35.
4. *Hippocrates*, translated by W. H. S. Jones; quoted in Coulter, *Divided Legacy I*, 26.
5. *Hippocrates*, translated by W. H. S. Jones; quoted in Coulter, *Divided Legacy I*, 79.
6. Coulter, *Divided Legacy I*, 196.
7. Coulter, *Divided Legacy I*, 76.
8. Aulus Cornelius Celsus, *De Medicina*; quoted in Coulter, *Divided Legacy I*, 274.
9. Aulus Cornelius Celsus, *Prooemium*; quoted in Coulter, *Divided Legacy I*, 252.
10. Aulus Cornelius Celsus, *Aphorisms*; quoted in Coulter, *Divided Legacy I*, 256.
11. Aulus Cornelius Celsus, *De Medicina*; quoted in Coulter, *Divided Legacy I*, 258.
12. Galen; quoted in Coulter, *Divided Legacy I*, 308.
13. Paracelsus, *Das Erste Buch der Grossen Wundarznei*; quoted in Coulter, *Divided Legacy I*, 346.
14. Paracelsus, *Intimatio, Basileae, 5 Juni 1527*; quoted in Coulter, *Divided Legacy I*, 347.

15. Paracelsus, *Entwuerfe zu den vier Buecher des Opus Paramirum*; quoted in Coulter, *Divided Legacy I*, 380.
16. Paracelsus, *Das Buch Paragranum*; quoted in Coulter, *Divided Legacy I*, 425.
17. Coulter, *Divided Legacy I*, 384.
18. Paracelsus, *Liber de podagricis et suis speciebus*; quoted in Coulter, *Divided Legacy I*, 417.
19. Paracelsus, *Drei Buecher der Wundarznei*; quoted in Coulter, *Divided Legacy I*, 426.
20. Paracelsus; quoted in *Doctrine of Signatures, Io Magazine 5*, Ann Arbor, Michigan, 1968: 4.
21. Paracelsus, *Von Oeffnung der Haut*; quoted in Coulter, *Divided Legacy I*, 443.
22. Oswald Croll, "Preface Concerning Signatures"; quoted in *Doctrine of Signatures*, op. cit., 31–32.
23. Harris L. Coulter, *Divided Legacy, A History of the Schism in Medical Thought, Volume II: Progress and Regress: J. B. Van Helmont to Claude Bernard* (Berkeley, California: North Atlantic Books, 1988), 110–11.
24. Jan Baptista Van Helmont, *Oriatrike, or Physick Refined (1662)*; quoted in Coulter, *Divided Legacy II*, 15.
25. Ibid., 33.
26. Ibid., 56.
27. William Harvey, *The Works of William Harvey (1847)*; quoted in Coulter, *Divided Legacy II*, 129.
28. Thomas Steele Hall, *Rene Descartes: Treatise of Man* (Cambridge: Harvard, 1972), 5–6.
29. Hermann Boerhaave, *Dr. Boerhaave's Academical Lectures on the Theory of Physic, Being a Genuine Translation of his Institutes and Explanatory Comment (1742–1746)*; quoted in Coulter, *Divided Legacy II*, 130.
30. Coulter, *Divided Legacy II*, 171.
31. Giorgio Baglivi, *De Praxi Medica ad Priscam Observandi Rationem Revocanda Libri Duo (1696)*; quoted in Coulter, *Divided Legacy II*, 185.
32. Thomas Sydenham, *The Works of Thomas Sydenham (1848–1850)*; quoted in Coulter, *Divided Legacy II*, 187.
33. Ibid., 191.
34. Théophile de Bordeu, *Oeuvres (1818)*; quoted in Coulter, *Divided Legacy II*, 241–42.

Chapter Three

1. James Tyler Kent, *Lectures on Homoeopathic Philosophy (1900)*, republished by North Atlantic Books (Berkeley, California: 1979), 39.
2. Claude Bernard, *An Introduction to the Study of Experimental Medicine* (New York: Dover, 1957).

3. Walter B. Cannon, *The Wisdom of the Body* (New York: Norton, 1942).

4. Hans Selye, *The Stress of Life* (New York: McGraw-Hill, 1978), 12.

5. Ilya Prigogine and Isabelle Stengers, *Order Out of Chaos* (New York: Bantam, 1984).

6. Ullman, "Homeopathic Medicine."
   [2–5 quoted in Ullman]

7. Edward Whitmont, *The Alchemy of Healing: Psyche and Soma* (Berkeley, California: North Atlantic Books, 1993), 105.

8. Samuel Hahnemann, *The Organon of Medicine;* quoted in Harris L. Coulter, *Divided Legacy, Volume II: The Origins of Modern Western Medicine* (Berkeley, California: North Atlantic Books, 1988), 385–86.

9. Ibid., 12.

10. George Vithoulkas, *The Science of Homeopathy: A Modern Textbook,* Volume I (Athens, Greece: A.S.O.H.M., 1978), 134–35.

11. See Harris L. Coulter, *AIDS and Syphilis: The Hidden Link* (Berkeley, California: North Atlantic Books, 1987).

12. Samuel Hahnemann, *The Lesser Writings;* quoted in Harris L. Coulter, *Divided Legacy II,* 375.

13. M. L. Tyler, *Homoeopathic Drug Pictures* (Holsworthy Devon, England: Health Science Press, 1942).

14. Samuel Hahnemann, *The Organon of Medicine;* quoted in Coulter, *Divided Legacy II,* 350.

15. Claude Lévi-Strauss, *Totemism,* trans. from the French by Rodney Needham (Boston: Beacon Press, 1963).

16. Edward P. Tine, Sr., "Repertory of the Homoeopathic Materia Medica" (Washington, D. C.: *Journal of the American Institute of Homeopathy,* Vol. 58, No. 1–2, Jan.–Feb., 1965).

17. Didier Grandgeorge, M. D., *The Spirit of Homeopathic Medicines: Essential Insights to 300 Remedies,* translated from the French by Juliana Barnard (Berkeley, California: North Atlantic Books, 1998), 205.

18. Tyler, *Homoeopathic Drug Pictures,* 707–16; Grandgeorge, *The Spirit of Homeopathic Medicines,* 165.

19. Tyler, *Homoeopathic Drug Pictures,* 143–52; Grandgeorge, *The Spirit of Homeopathic Medicines,* 47.

20. Samuel Hahnemann; quoted in Tyler, *Homoeopathic Drug Pictures,* 147.

21. Tyler, *Homoeopathic Drug Pictures,* 798–801; Grandgeorge, *The Spirit of Homeopathic Medicines,* 187–88.

22. Tyler, *Homoeopathic Drug Pictures,* 289–99.

23. Grandgeorge, *The Spirit of Homeopathic Medicines,* 67.

24. Tyler, *Homoeopathic Drug Pictures,* 586–93; Grandgeorge, *The Spirit of Homeopathic Medicines,* 138–39.

25. Tine, Sr., "Repertory of the Homoeopathic Materia Medica."

26. Tyler, *Homoeopathic Drug Pictures*, 666–70; Grandgeorge, *The Spirit of Homeopathic Medicines*, 156–57.

27. W. A. Boyson, "Repertory of the Homoeopathic Materia Medica" (Washington, D. C.: *Journal of the American Institute of Homeopathy*, Vol. 58, No. 1–2, Jan.–Feb., 1965).

28. Philip M. Bailey, M. D., *Homeopathic Psychology: Personality Profiles of the Major Constitutional Remedies* (Berkeley, California: North Atlantic Books, 1995), 279–84; Tyler, *Homoeopathic Drug Pictures*, 681–87; Grandgeorge, *The Spirit of Homeopathic Medicines*, 159–61.

29. Ibid.

30. Tyler, *Homoeopathic Drug Pictures*, 683.

31. Ibid., 830.

32. Bailey, *Homeopathic Psychology: Personality Profiles of the Major Constitutional Remedies*, 386–97.

33. Grandgeorge, *The Spirit of Homeopathic Medicines*, 192; Tyler, *Homoeopathic Drug Pictures*, 830–42; Bailey, *Homeopathic Psychology: Personality Profiles of the Major Constitutional Remedies*, 386–88.

34. Grandgeorge, *The Spirit of Homeopathic Medicines*, 194.

35. Samuel Hahnemann, *The Organon of Medicine;* quoted in Kent, op. cit.

36. Jonathan Shore, "After the Remedy," undated sheet given to patients.

37. Theodore Enslin, speaking at a seminar at Goddard College, Plainfield, Vermont, May 1977.

38. Kent, *Lectures*, 253–65.

39. Whitmont, *The Alchemy of Healing*, ix.

40. See Harris Coulter, *Vaccination, Social Violence, and Criminality: The Medical Assault on the American Brain* (Berkeley, California: North Atlantic Books, 1990).

41. Theodore Enslin, speaking at a seminar at Goddard College, Plainfield, Vermont, May 1977.

42. Whitmont, *The Alchemy of Healing*, 10.

43. Hahnemann, *The Lesser Writings;* quoted in Coulter, *Divided Legacy II*, 389.

44. Whitmont, *The Alchemy of Healing*, 75.

45. G. P. Barnard and James H. Stephenson, "Microdose Paradox: A New Biophysical Concept" (Washington, D. C.: *Journal of the American Institute of Homeopathy*, Sept.–Oct., 1967), 278.

46. Ibid.

47. Whitmont, *The Alchemy of Healing*, 6.

48. Gorman, "Take a Little Deadly Nightshade...," 73.

49. Jonathan Shore, personal communication, 1998.

50. Whitmont, *The Alchemy of Healing*, 7.

51. Ibid., 139–40.

52. Gorman, "Take a Little Deadly Nightshade...," 28.

53. E. Davenas et al., *Nature* (June 30, 1988), 816–18.
54. J. Maddox et al., *Nature* (July 28, 1988), 287–90.
55. David Concar, "'Ghost Molecules' Theory Back from the Dead," *New Scientist* (March 16, 1991), 10.
56. Jacques Benveniste et al., "L'agitation de solutions hautement dilués n'induit pas d'activité biologique spécifique," *Comptes Rendus del Academie des Sciences Paris, 312* (série II), (1991), 461–66.
57. Ullman, "Homeopathic Medicine."
[53–56 quoted in Ullman]
58. Robert Poole, "More Squabbling Over Unbelievable Results," *Science* (August 15, 1988), Vol. 241: 658.
59. Thomas H. Maugh II, "Journal Probe of Lab Test Results Sparks Furor," *The Los Angeles Times*, July 27, 1988.
60. K. C. Cole, *Sympathetic Vibrations* (New York: Bantam, 1985), 265.
61. M. V. Singer et al., "Low Concentrations of Ethanol Stimulate Gastric Secretion Independent of Gastrin Release in Humans," *Gastroenterology 85* (1985), 1254.
62. Ullman, "Homeopathic Medicine."
[60 and 61 quoted in Ullman]
63. Kent, *Lectures*, 96.
64. Theodore Enslin, speaking at a seminar at Goddard College, Plainfield, Vermont, May 1977.
65. Wyrth P. Baker, Allen C. Neiswander, and W. W. Young, *Introduction to Homoeotherapeutics* (Washington, D.C.: American Institute of Homeopathy, 1974).
66. Gorman, "Take a Little Deadly Nightshade. . .," 28.
67. Dana Ullman, "Extremely Dilute Solutions Create Unique Stable Ice Crystals in Room-Temperature Water—Implications for Medicine, Manufacturing, and Technology," press release (Berkeley, California: Homeopathic Educational Services, http://www.homeopathic.com, December 29, 1997).
68. Ibid.
69. Ibid. [See also Shui-Yin Lo, Ph.D., "Physical Properties of Water with I_E Structures," *Modern Physics Letters B*, 10, 19 (1996): 921–30.]
70. Edward Whitmont, "Toward a Basic Law of Psychic and Somatic Interrelationship," *The Homeopathic Recorder* (February 1949), 206.
71. Carl Jung, *Psychology and Alchemy*, trans. from the German by R.F.C. Hull (London: Routledge & Kegan Paul, 1953), 132.
72. Whitmont, *Alchemy of Healing* (Berkeley, California: North Atlantic Books, 1993), 216.
73. Edward Whitmont, "The Analysis of a Dynamic Totality: *Sepia*," *The Homeopathic Recorder*, reprint, 1948–1955, 232.
74. Ibid., 233.

75. Edward Whitmont, "Natrum Muriaticum," *The Homeopathic Recorder* (1948), 119.
76. Edward Whitmont, "Phosphor," *The Homeopathic Recorder* (April 1949), 265.
77. Rudolf Hauschka, *The Nature of Substance,* trans. from the German by Mary T. Richards and Marjorie Spock (London: Stuart and Watkins, 1968), 136–37.
78. Edward Whitmont, "Lycopodium: A Psychosomatic Study," *The Homeopathic Recorder* (1948): 264–65.
79. Edward Whitmont, "Psycho-physiological Reflections on Lachesis," *British Homeopathic Recorder,* January 1975.
80. Edward Whitmont, "Non-causality as a Unifying Principle of Psychosomatics—Sulphur," *Psyche and Substance* (Berkeley, California: North Atlantic Books, 1991), 147–55.
   All of the Edward Whitmont articles are republished in updated form in *Psyche and Substance: Essays on Homeopathy in the Light of Jungian Psychology* (Berkeley: North Atlantic Books, 1992).
81. Stanley Keleman, personal communication, 1978.

Chapter Four

I have reconstructed Samuel Hahnemann's biography primarily from Richard Haehl, *Samuel Hahnemann, His Life and Work,* Volume I (London: Homeopathic Publishing Company, 1922). General information from the text will not be cited but specific quotations will.

1. Haehl, *Samuel Hahnemann,* 10.
2. Ibid., 11.
3. Ibid., 36.
4. Ibid., 35.
5. Ibid., 58.
6. Ibid., 63.
7. Ibid., 64.
8. Samuel Hahnemann, *Organon der rationellen Heilkunde* (Dresden, 1810), trans. by C. E. Wheeler, *Organon of the Rational Art of Healing* (London, 1913), 18. Quoted in Rima Handley, *A Homeopathic Love Story: The Story of Samuel and Mélanie Hahnemann* (Berkeley, California: North Atlantic Books, 1990).
9. Ibid., 20.
10. Ibid., 322.
11. R. E. Dudgeon (ed.), *Lesser Writings of Samuel Hahnemann* (New York: William Radde, 1852), 823.
12. Ibid.
13. Ibid., 819.

14. Ibid., 822.
15. Ibid., 859.
    [11–15 quoted in Handley]
16. G. P. Barnard and James H. Stephenson, "Microdose Paradox: A New Biophysical Concept," 279.
17. Haehl, *Samuel Hahnemann*, 126.
18. Coulter, *Divided Legacy*, Volume II, 170.
19. Ibid., 171.
20. Gorman, "Take a Little Deadly Nightshade...," 28.
21. Quoted in Haehl, *Samuel Hahnemann*, 100.
22. Dudgeon, *Lesser Writings*, 712–15. Quoted in Handley.
23. Handley, *A Homeopathic Love Story*, 76–77.
24. Haehl, *Samuel Hahnemann*, 110. Quoted in Handley.
25. Handley, *A Homeopathic Love Story*, 77–78.
26. Samuel Hahnemann, *The Chronic Diseases, Their Peculiar Nature, and Their Homeopathic Cure* (Philadelphia: Boericke & Tafel, 1904), 12.
27. Ibid.
28. Ibid., 38.
29. Samuel Hahnemann, *The Chronic Diseases*, second edition (1835), trans. by L. Tafel (Philadelphia: Boericke & Tafel, 1896), 81. Quoted in Handley, *A Homeopathic Love Story*, 83–84.
30. Haehl, *Samuel Hahnemann*, 179.
31. Ibid.
32. Personal letters quoted in Handley, *A Homeopathic Love Story*, 5–6.
33. Haehl, *Samuel Hahnemann*, 222.
34. Handley, *A Homeopathic Love Story*, 6.
35. Haehl, *Samuel Hahnemann*, Volume II, 328. Quoted in Handley, *A Homeopathic Love Story*, 12.

Chapter Five

1. Coulter, *Divided Legacy*, Volume III, 62–63.
2. Ibid., 168.
3. Ibid.
4. Ibid., 180.
5. Ibid., 106.
6. Haehl, *Samuel Hahnemann*, 187.
7. Coulter, *Divided Legacy III*, 264–65.
8. Ibid., 269–70.
9. Ibid., 403.
10. Ibid., 411.
11. Ibid., 414.
12. Ibid., 438.

13. Ibid., 441.
14. Ibid., 447–48.
15. Gorman, "Take a Little Deadly Nightshade...," 26.
16. Mark Twain, "A Majestic Literary Fossil," *Harper's Magazine* (February 1890): 444.
17. D. Reilly et al., "Is Homoeopathy a Placebo Response? Controlled Trial of Homoeopathic Potency with Pollen in Hayfever as Model," *Lancet* (October 18, 1986): 881–86.
18. R.G. Gibson et al., "Homoeopathic Therapy in Rheumatoid Arthritis: Evaluation by Double-Blind Clinical Therapeutic Trial," *British Journal of Clinical Pharmacology 9* (1980): 453–59.
19. A.M. Scofield, "Experimental Research in Homoeopathy: A Critical Review," *British Homoeopathic Journal 73* (July–October 1984): 161–80, 211–26.
20. J.C. Cazin et al., "A Study of the Effects of Decimal and Centesimal Dilution of Arsenic on Retention and Mobilization of Arsenic in the Rat," *Human Toxicology* (July 1987): 315–20.
21. J. Paterson, "Report on Mustard Gas Experiments," *Journal of the American Institute of Homeopathy 37* (1944): 47–50, 88–92.
22. W.E. Boyd, "The Action of Microdoses of Mercuric Chloride on Diastase," *British Homoeopathic Journal 31* (1941): 1–28; Vol. 32 (1942): 106–11.
23. L.M. Singh and G. Gupta, "Antiviral Efficacy of Homoeopathic Drugs Against Animal Viruses," *British Homoeopathic Journal 74* (July 1985): 168–74.
24. K. Khanna and S. Chandra, "Control of Guava Fruit Rot Caused by Pestaolotia Psidii with Homeopathic Drugs," *Plant Dis. Rep. 61* (1977): 362; "A Homeopathic Drug Controls Mango Fruit Rot Caused by Pestaolotia Mangiferae," *Experientia 34* (1978): 1167.
25. Ullman, "Homeopathic Medicine."
[17–24 quoted from Ullman, op. cit.]
26. Ullman, personal communication, 1997.
27. Gorman, "Take a Little Deadly Nightshade...," 23.

Index